Health Expert: W

For years, allopathic medicine has treated menopause as a disease brought on by a deficiency of hormones, instead of a perfectly natural bodily transition. *Secrets of a Natural Menopause* will help you discover what's best for *your* body and empower you to take control of your own health and well-being.

Herbs for menopause: How safe are herbs? ... how to make tinctures, salves, etc. ... how to fill gelatin capsules ... what herbs do ... how to choose the herbal properties you need ... all about Dong Quai, wonder herb for women ... garlic: what scientists say

Vitamins and minerals for menopause: How and when to take supplements ... how many carrots equal a dose? ... vitamin and mineral terms ... food and herbal sources of vitamins and minerals

Homeopathy for menopause: How to take homeopathic medicine ... where to get homeopathic remedies

Foods for menopause: Health tips for a happy menopause ... fiber facts and figures ... vegetable combining for complete proteins

Yoga for menopause: How to practice Yoga ... some Yoga poses ... suggested Yoga routines

One benefit of these effective, drug-free methods of alleviating the emotional, mental, and physical symptoms of menopause is that using them may help you avoid the increased risk of developing certain cancers that have been linked to estrogen replacement therapy.

Menopause is no more a disease than is puberty—it is simply another phase of life. Find out what is best for your body and your transition, and become your own health expert for a very important clientele of one: you.

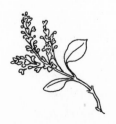

About the Author

Edna Copeland Ryneveld, who was born and raised in Texas, now lives in Bolivar, Missouri, where she operates a health food store. She has been a teacher and worked as a secretary in physics research and aerospace in California, and also has been a copywriter and traffic director for a Bolivar radio station. She prefers living in the slow lane, running the health food store, and writing. In addition to her first book for Llewellyn, *Transits in Reverse,* she has contributed to *Sacred Sites,* and has other books in the works. Her poetry and articles have appeared in national magazines.

To Write to the Author

If you wish to contact the author or would like more information about this book, please write to the author in care of Llewellyn Worldwide and we will forward your request. Both the author and publisher appreciate hearing from you and learning of your enjoyment of this book and how it has helped you. Llewellyn Worldwide cannot guarantee that every letter written to the author can be answered, but all will be forwarded. Please write to:

Edna Ryneveld
c/o Llewellyn Worldwide
P.O. Box 64383-K596, St. Paul, MN 55164-0383, U.S.A.

Please enclose a self-addressed, stamped envelope for reply, or $1.00 to cover costs.
If outside U.S.A., enclose international postal reply coupon.

Free Catalog From Llewellyn Worldwide

For more than 90 years Llewellyn has brought its readers knowledge in the fields of metaphysics and human potential. Learn about the newest books in spiritual guidance, natural healing, astrology, occult philosophy, and more. Enjoy book reviews, new age articles, a calendar of events, plus current advertised products and services. To get your free copy of *Llewellyn's New Worlds of Mind and Spirit,* send your name and address to:

Llewellyn's New Worlds of Mind and Spirit
P.O. Box 64383-K596, St. Paul, MN 55164-0383, U.S.A.

Llewellyn's Health and Healing Series

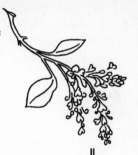

Secrets of a Natural Menopause

A Positive Drug-Free Approach

Edna Copeland Ryneveld

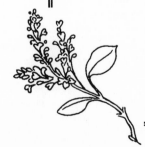

1994
Llewellyn Publications
St. Paul, Minnesota 55164-0383, U.S.A.

FIRST EDITION
First Printing

Cover art by Lucy Synk
Interior illustrations by Lisa Hunt
Editing and interior design by Connie Hill

Library of Congress Cataloging-in-publication Data
Ryneveld, Edna Copeland
    Secrets of a natural menopause : a positive drug-free approach /
  Edna Copeland Ryneveld.
      p.   cm. — (Llewellyn's health and healing series)
  Includes bibliographical references and index.
  ISBN 1-56718-596-7
  1. Menopause—Complications—Alternative treatment.   I. Title. II. Series.
  RG186.R96   1994
  618.1'75—dc20   94-33401
                                                                   CIP

Llewellyn Publications
A Division of Llewellyn Worldwide, Ltd.
P.O. Box 64383, St. Paul, MN 55164-0383

Dedication

To all women on the Great Journey of Integration
and to my Crystal Garden friends in particular,
I dedicate this book.

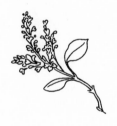

Warning

The remedies, recipes, and suggestions in this book are for your information only, for consideration in your pursuit of complete self-responsibility. Neither the author nor the pubisher is responsible for any effects of any procedure listed herein.

Consult your inner guide before deciding on any form of self-treatment. *We also strongly suggest you consult a holistic physician for advice before self-treating any serious ailment.*

Table of Contents

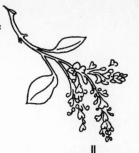

PREFACE

Menopause—A Seeding

> *The mark of your ignorance is the depth of your belief in injustice and tragedy. What the caterpillar calls the end of the world, the master calls a butterfly.*
> —Richard Bach
> *Illusions*

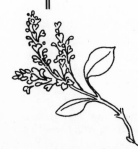

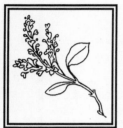 It may seem odd that I refer to what most people think of as the last stage of a woman's life as a seeding, but I like to think of menopause as a beginning, a birth of the spiritual wise woman, who has been struggling and gestating within for so long. Now she is birthing herself, and, though yet in her infancy, has much to offer those who follow.

Consider this: seeds burst forth only from flowers which, despite many possible trials, tribulations, and hazards, have survived—an obvious statement, but an important one, contemplated in terms of evolution. Embodying much more than the physical means to the next generation, the seeds of such flowers are compact treasure troves of knowledge. The information jewels of the plant kingdom, these seeds can grow to imprint their own seeds with their own pearls of wisdom gleaned from experience. They do this without having to laboriously reexperience and reprogram everything themselves. Very efficiently, wisdom and knowledge are not demeaned or ignored simply because they come from an "old" plant.

As it is with the "pearls" of the mature plant, so it is with the accumulated wisdom and knowledge of the mature woman entering a new phase of life known as menopause. There is much to be learned from such a woman. Or so it should be.

Unfortunately, in youth-oriented western societies, aging bodies and minds—especially of women—are devalued.

Not coincidentally, it is only in these societies that the term "menopause" and the event itself have negative connotations and negative health symptoms. In a 150-nation study of menopause, negative symptoms were most prevalent where women lost power and mobility as they aged.[1] The study found that in other areas, such as Pakistan, where women

---

1 John B. McKinlay and Sonja M. McKinlay, "Depression in Middle-Aged Women: Social Circumstances versus Estrogen Deficiency," *The Psychology of Women,* Mary Walsh, editor, New Haven: Yale University Press, 1987, pp. 158–159.

have many taboos and restrictions during their childbearing years, but have more freedom and authority after menopause, negative menopausal symptoms were nil. There are even variations within the United States: African-American women have fewer menopausal symptoms than Jewish women. Biological differences could be postulated, but there is no evidence for this. It is, however, interesting to note the differences in the respect and power accorded older women in these two groups. The correlation is exact.

The conclusion is inescapable. Our attitudes and beliefs condition our bodily responses. Attitudes and beliefs can be changed. You need not buy into "thin, young, and non-gray is best and most beautiful." Change your attitudes and beliefs, and your body will respond. Conversely, change your body and you change your attitudes and beliefs. You can become not only healthier, but also more vibrant, effective, and self-confident, as an aura of glowing beauty and innate authority surrounds you.

Changing attitudes is a process that may take some time, they are so well ingrained in most of us; and, for whatever reasons (today's stress levels can be one), many women do experience uncomfortable, and sometimes distressing, symptoms during menopause. This book gives you many possible routes to freedom from these symptoms. These different routes, reported as effective over many years' (sometimes thousands of years) experience by women of all nations, by herbalists, by grannies, by "ancient Chinese," and by scientists, let you choose the method best for you.

The first step is for we women to take control of our own bodies and to expend some of our vast nurturing abilities on ourselves. We must toss out the idea that only experts know what is good for us. Listen to the wise women who have gone before us. Listen. Can you hear them? They are whispering to your own inner wise woman that, as we are of the earth, the gentle ways of the herbs and stones are best; as we are of spirit, the ways of the breath and unseen energies of the air and cosmos are best; as we are of mind, the ways of the third eye and our "other" ears are best; and as we are the seeds of our ancestors and the seeds for all who follow, the ways of our own hearts are best.

Listen to your developing wise woman, and you'll unerringly choose the proper treatment for your own body's transformation from among the many ways brought together for you in this book.

You may choose from among several alternative healing—or, as I prefer—"healthing" methods. You may go one route exclusively or combine several. Bear in mind that your body is unique and you may or may not respond to a particular method or product exactly the same as Aunt Jane, your next-door neighbor, the participants in a scientific study, or all those millions of ancient Chinese.

There is but one caveat: Begin cautiously, especially when ingesting or applying any substance, no matter how natural it may be. Contrary to Mae West's famous comment, too much of a good thing *does* sometimes fall short of wonderful. You can overdose even on water; and anyone can be allergic to anything.

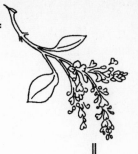

CHAPTER 1

Herbs for Menopause

If we bless our bodies, our bodies will bless us.

—Gloria Steinem

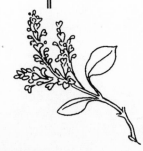

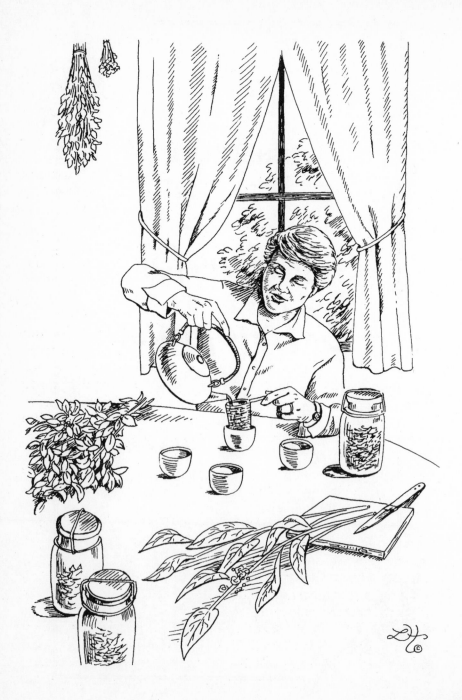

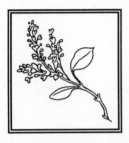 Weeds—otherwise known as herbs when you value them—are potent little health factories right under your nose; friends who can help to heal your wounds and your illnesses; friends who can help you over the rough spots in your life or comfort you every day, just by being there. How much better this is than devitalized, overprocessed, and transshipped foods which actually stress our bodies, giving them so little nourishment they can barely function, let alone be vibrantly healthy.

Filled with fat and calories, but essentially undernourished nonetheless, our bodies crave more food. Responding to our body's needs, we then stuff in more addicting and devitalized foods. Under the circumstances, our bodies hold out remarkably well for a time, but inevitably illness and degeneration result, and we blame them on aging. Then we end up taking drugs to quell the symptoms and illnesses that occur. The drugs themselves then put us under additional, though different, stresses, which then require more drugs to temper *those* symptoms, which . . . well, it's an endless cycle.

By contrast, when herbs are used to nourish and/or to treat our selves, we come once again into alignment with the universal energies natural and familiar to our bodies.

Synthesizing the vibrations of fire, water (sunlight and moonlight), earth, and air, herbs convert these energies into a form that we can utilize. Oriental herbalists maintain that herbs assist the body's natural healing process because they supply what is missing from the patient's energy field, thus bringing about a balance of energies and "curing" the person. A western scientist would say that garlic, for instance, contains an agent which kills germs and viruses and *that* is why, when you took it, you got over your cold or bladder infection. Native Americans urge that we honor and respect the life force in all living things to prevent our hearts from becoming hardened, and thus ultimately losing respect for our fellow humans, as well. Respect for the inherent powers within herbs, they say, allows us to derive the most benefit from them, and it is true. Attitude plays a large role in our health and the assistance we may receive from any particular healing method. (Many people recover from placebos alone!) Herbs should not be popped like aspirin.

Nor should we ridicule the power of ritual in eliciting respect and cooperation from our own body and from the herbs themselves, even if the ritual is no more than our own tea ceremony and a calm demeanor of expectation that the herb will help us in some way, and of gratitude for its gentle healing properties.

Whatever the terminology—whether it's energy balancing or chemical warfare, the bottom line is that herbs do benefit us, both as food and as medicines. They always have.

ARTHRITIS/JOINT PROBLEMS

Some form of arthritis or joint problem is reported by about 48 percent of women as a symptom of menopause. Arthritis can be greatly helped, even cured, by many natural products, including herbs, foods, vitamins, minerals, and exercises. The problem is there are many different kinds of arthritis and even more different kinds of people. What may be just the thing for one person may be of no use to another, so the trick is finding the natural treatment that helps *your* arthritis.

Arthritis is a condition said by many to be the result of impure blood and resulting toxicity throughout the body's organs. A class of herbs termed "alteratives" (they alter, that is, purify the blood) is therefore recommended by herbalists for arthritis and a number of other conditions, including cancer. Alteratives should be taken over a long period of time to slowly cleanse the body of impurities. (Quick detoxing can be very nasty and unpleasant!) Of course, poor diet and other bad habits should be eliminated to aid the body in detoxification. It doesn't help to keep piling dirt in faster than herbal assistance can shovel it out.

Whatever you do, don't give up. In most cases, you cannot expect an overnight miracle with natural remedies—they work by aiding your body to heal itself—give them time to help. It probably took you many years to develop your condition; it will also take time to get rid of it. Keeping individual differences in mind, if a particular herb doesn't result in improvement after, say, several months, then try another. Keep searching. Put your desire for assistance out into the Universe; ask; *something* will be just what you need, and you *will* find it.

❧ The following is an herbal combination helpful for many problems in addition to arthritis, including so-called age spots, mainly because it is such a capable liver purifier: 4 parts CHAPARRAL[1], 2 parts YUCCA, 1 part BLACK COHOSH, 1 part DANDELION, 1 part SASSAFRAS, 1 part PRICKLY ASH BARK, 1 part GINGER ROOT, 1 part BURDOCK ROOT. Mix the individual herbs, powder them with a blender or mortar and pestle, and put into double-ought (#00) capsules (see Chapter 2, Herbal Notebook). A dosage of two capsules, three times a day, is useful. By paying attention to your own responses, your intuition, or by kinetic testing (see Herbal Notebook), you can determine your personal optimum dosage. Adjust it over time, as you improve.

❧ DANDELION, CHICKWEED, YUCCA, DEVIL'S CLAW, and BURDOCK seeds, roots, or leaves are also used successfully in the treatment of arthritis. These may be taken in capsules or used in infusions individually (see Herbal Notebook), or you may mix in any combination you desire. BURDOCK seed tea is also an excellent choice in the treatment of gout, because it increases the urinary output of uric acid, as does DEVIL'S CLAW, CELERY SEED, or CORN SILK tea.

❧ CHICKWEED added to bath water brings relief from joint pain and sore muscles. Twenty or thirty drops of a tincture made from the fresh plant (see Herbal Notebook) taken in water two or three times a day for several months will also do wonders for your joints, as will eating fresh CHICKWEED or drinking CHICKWEED tea daily.

❧ ALFALFA, an Arabic word meaning "father of all herbs," is also beneficial for arthritis. Six tablets or capsules taken three times a day has been the dosage necessary for several people I know. Drinking ALFALFA tea is useful, too.

❧ As little as a teaspoon of (powdered) SEAWEED (KELP, DULSE, etc.) a day has been found helpful for gout, arthritic pain, and all sorts of menopausal symptoms. SEAWEED is a floating powerhouse of nutrition and a great little hormone balancer. (I like one-half teaspoon of powdered kelp stirred into a glass of grapefruit juice twice a day to accompany my herbs and vitamins.

---

1 Chaparral has been banned by the FDA recently, due to what they termed "liver problems." This extremely cleansing herb must be used with adequate care and intelligence for it to be safe—as it has been utilized to great healing effect for hundreds, if not thousands, of years. See Chapter 2, "How Safe are Herbs."

ஃ Several companies have herbal combinations, already mixed and encapsulated, which have traditionally helped arthritis and similar problems. These include Nature's Way's YuccaAR™ and Red Clover Combination™.

ஃ HORSETAIL, also known as SHAVEGRASS, helps to prevent arthritis and strengthens bones. It contains silicon in an easily assimilable form; very important for the osteoporosis-prone.

CONCEPTION

You cannot assume you're unable to get pregnant just because you haven't had a period for about six months. At menopause, ovulation slows down considerably and can be erratic before it actually stops for good. After one year with no periods, especially after age 52, the chance that you will conceive is extremely small, but is still not impossible.

CONTRACEPTION

ஃ Certain herbs and foods (see Chapter 7) contain substances known as phytoestrogens. High levels of this compound may inhibit fertility (while, incidentally, providing protection from breast and ovarian cancers), according to Claude L. Hughes, Jr., M.D., Ph.D., of Duke University.[2] He found that vegetarians have phytoestrogen levels 100 times higher than those who eat the Standard American Diet (SAD). A diet low in phytoestrogen has been linked with reproductive-system cancers in both men and women (as well as heart disease). It is speculated that including herbs and foods high in phytoestrogens in the daily diet of menopausal and postmenopausal women might reduce the risk of developing these chronic diseases. Some herbs containing phytoestrogens include: ALFALFA, ANISE, RED CLOVER, FENNEL, GARLIC, HOPS, LICORICE ROOT, OATS, PARSLEY, and SAGE.

ஃ BLUE COHOSH, *Caulophyllum thalictroides*, also known as "SQUAW-ROOT," an emmenagogue, may be used to promote and regulate menses. It is reported that the Chippewas used a strong decoction of the root as a contraceptive.[3] It is not taken when pregnant, unless one

---

2 Simpkins, Deborah, "Duke Researcher Says Plant Compounds Can Affect Women's Health," *Duke University News*, Jan. 29, 1992; and McKeown, L. A., "Diet High in Fruits and Vegetables Linked to Lower Breast Cancer Risk," *Medical Tribune*, July 9, 1992.

3 *Hygieia*, Jeannine Parvati, Freestone Innerprizes, Felton, CA, 1978, p. 24.

wants to induce labor. It is said to promote a rapid and painless delivery. It could, therefore, be used early on as an abortifacient.

❦ A daily infusion of the flower tops of BLESSED THISTLE, *Onicus benedictus*, is also reported to be contraceptive. It can be an abortifacient, too; many herbal texts say it should not be taken in quantity if pregnant.

❦ JUNIPER, *Juniperus communis L.*, an emmenagogue said, as well, to be temporarily contraceptive if the berries are made into a tea and drunk for three consecutive days.

❦ WILD YAM root, *Dioscorea villosa*, is another contraceptive. It contains the basic raw ingredients that were synthesized and made into "The Pill." Take three capsules morning and night for two months before you rely on it alone, for as long as you want to avoid conception. There are no harmful side effects. It is also very calming, will normalize menstruation, relieve cramps, and alleviate ulcers and gas.

❦ PENNYROYAL has been used both as a contraceptive and as an abortifacient. Some report drinking one cup of PENNYROYAL infusion a day as a preventative. As a rule, one should not exceed three cups per day.

CONSTIPATION

Over a third of menopausal women report experiencing constipation. Many herbs have been used traditionally for their laxative effects, either as teas, capsules, or as food. You should be aware, though, that, except for the food items and bulking agents listed below, prolonged use of any laxative, no matter how natural, should be avoided. They are not addicting, as are, say, tobacco or cocaine, but if your bowel muscles come to depend on laxatives to do their work for them, they'll get lazy and won't want to work on their own (just like any other unused muscle).

❦ CHICKWEED, great as a salad or in a salad if you can get it (it grows wild in many areas of the country), or take as tea or in capsules.

❦ YERBA MATÉ, or just MATÉ (pronounced mah-TAY), as a tea.

❦ DANDELION, as an infusion of the fresh root.

❦ NETTLE leaves, as a tea after dinner or, if you can get NETTLE fresh, use it juiced or as cooked greens daily, or at least several times a week for several weeks.

🎗 OATMEAL, consumed as part of the daily diet (great for bones and nerves, too) or OATSTRAW tea taken daily.

🎗 OREGON GRAPE ROOT is good for chronic constipation. Make a decoction and take 3 ounces before meals. This should be made fresh daily; or use a tincture, 30 to 60 drops in water, also three times daily.

🎗 CASCARA SAGRADA, usually taken in capsule form.

🎗 SENNA leaves, as tea, tablet, or capsule. Do not use senna if you have piles, prolapsed intestine, or inflammation anywhere in the intestinal tract. It is a stimulant laxative; therefore DO NOT USE DURING PREGNANCY.

🎗 APPLES, preferably raw, at least one daily; other fruits and vegetables, as many raw as is practical.

🎗 WHOLE GRAINS daily.

🎗 FIBER and WATER and EXERCISE are the best laxatives you can find.

🎗 PECTIN, as tablet or capsule, or just eat plenty of APPLES.

🎗 PSYLLIUM (pronounced SIL-ly-um) seed or husks, a bulking agent that increases the water in the bowels, thereby assisting evacuation. CAUTION: You MUST drink plenty of water when taking PSYLLIUM or any other bulking agent. It should not be taken at the same time you take other supplements, as it impedes their digestion (it forms an indigestible mass). Also: Do not take if you have a bowel obstruction or perforation.

🎗 BRAN, WHEAT or OAT, best when it is raw and unprocessed, is another bulking agent. Please read directions and cautions under "PSYLLIUM," above.

🎗 KELP,[4] about a teaspoonful (5 grams) of the powdered form daily, or use it as a salt substitute on your food (great on popcorn), or reconstitute dried SEAWEED and use it in cooking. You'll find suggestions in books on macrobiotic eating and on Japanese cooking.

🎗 Nature's Way's Naturalax #2™ is a good herbal combination laxative that helps to eliminate (over time) even old, impacted fecal matter. It consists of CASCARA SAGRADA BARK, BARBERRY ROOT BARK, CAYENNE, GINGER ROOT, GOLDENSEAL ROOT, LOBELIA, RED RASPBERRY LEAVES, TURKEY RHUBARB ROOT, and FENNEL SEED.

---

4 Powdered or granulated kelp contains 459 mg of sodium per tablespoon.

DEPRESSION, NERVES, LETHARGY, IRRITABILITY

Depression can be caused by anything from low blood sugar, to poor over-all nutrition, to high stress levels, to environmental pollutants, to hormone imbalance. In any case, many people have found the following herbs, alone or in combination, useful for depression. Remember, many herbs work slowly, helping the body to adjust and to rebuild itself. Give any herb a fair trial of at least a few weeks, ideally a few months. Don't let this discourage you. Many also report results in as few as three days.

❧ YERBA MATÉ (or MATÉ) infusion for lethargy.

❧ Also for lethargy, try a mix of DAMIANA, GOTU KOLA, ROSEMARY, and LAVENDER.

❧ DANDELION flower or leaf tea will soothe and nourish jangled nerves. Pour boiling water over a handful and steep a few minutes, adding honey, if you wish. CAUTION: Do not pick DANDELION leaves or flowers from chemically-treated lawns or along streets or roadsides.

❧ The following herbal combination provides calcium, a natural tranquilizer for relief of stress: COMFREY ROOT, ALFALFA, OAT STRAW, IRISH MOSS, HORSETAIL.

❧ Add a whole CLOVE or two to other teas, or a pinch of powdered CLOVES.

❧ DAMIANA, said to be a mild aphrodisiac for either sex, is also used for depression and as a nerve aid.

❧ SIBERIAN GINSENG tea or capsules.

❧ PAU D'ARCO tea or capsules.

❧ BLESSED THISTLE, tea or capsules.

❧ BLACK COHOSH root, as tea or capsules, is useful for all sorts of nervous conditions.

❧ SKULLCAP has been traditionally used to calm nerves and repair the nervous system, even repairing the spinal cord. Three ounces of infusion, three times a day, is a useful dose. SKULLCAP should be used in as fresh condition as possible.

❧ OAT groats, or even rolled OATS (OATMEAL), prepared as an infusion, tincture, fluid extract, or simply enjoyed as food, will help your nerves, restore some strength, and just generally help you cope.

✿ KELP, one teaspoon of the powder per day, or the equivalent (1000 mg.) in tablets or capsules. Soothes savage nerves.

✿ CAYENNE pepper, SIBERIAN GINSENG root, and GOTU KOLA combined, in capsules or as a tea, are a real picker-upper.

✿ GARLIC and ONIONS, eaten daily or, in the case of GARLIC, taken in odorless capsules, if you wish to spare your non-GARLIC-eating friends and coworkers. CAUTION: These members of the lily family contain sulfur and may not be tolerated by anyone allergic to sulfur.

✿ LICORICE ROOT, if blood sugar is suspected as the problem. Monitor yourself when taking it if you have high blood pressure, though.

✿ DANDELION root is also good for blood sugar regulation.

✿ MOTHERWORT, *Leonurus cardiaca*, herb will aid and soothe any number of nervous disturbances of menopause. CAUTION: It should not be used if pregnancy is suspected or if menstrual periods tend to be heavy. It can induce uterine bleeding.

✿ PUMPKIN SEEDS, containing tryptophan, will soothe nerves, relax you, and help you sleep. Dose: about six or seven ounces, nibbled and enjoyed.

✿ CHAMOMILE tea is very soothing and relaxing.

✿ PASSION FLOWER tea is wonderfully relaxing and calming. (It's also great for hyperactive grandchildren! So is CHAMOMILE and CAT-NIP.) It is likewise good for nerve debility and has even been useful for sciatica.

✿ CELERY SEED decoction is also soothing and relaxing to the nerves.

✿ CATNIP, tea or capsules, is relaxing and calming.

✿ PEPPERMINT, SPEARMINT, and VALERIAN root tea or capsules are also soothing and mellowing.

✿ SCHIZANDRA, *Schizandra chinensis*, an adaptogen from China and Tibet, is an energizer and antidepressant. CAUTION: It should be avoided by epileptics, people with high intracranial pressure or severe hypertension, and anyone with "high acidity."[5]

✿ WILD YAM ROOT is another calming herb.

---

5 *Herbal Healthline*, Vol. 2, No. 3, 1991.

EMOTIONS

You may find one, or any combination, of the herbs listed under Depression useful for "mysterious" mood swings. Experiment, be patient and observant. Or take the quick way: do muscle (kinetic) testing. (See Herbal Notebook.) During menopause, you can turn into a hormonal roller coaster, and your emotions may jump on for a ride. Some days (even some minutes!) everything may be on the upswing and all is right with the world. The next thing you know everything's downhill, and you're reaching for tissues in which to blow or the trusty iron skillet to throw. Kinetic testing allows you to determine what your body needs at the moment and even how much. Save the iron skillet for weight lifting.

In addition, the herbs and herbal combinations helpful for hormonal balancing may prevent or greatly alleviate symptoms of roller-coaster-itis.

ENDOMETRIOSIS

Menopause usually cures this condition, since it is sexual hormones that cause the errant uterine cells to produce the painful symptoms. If you're not too far from menopause and the symptoms are not life-threatening or debilitating, you might want to talk with your doctor about postponing the hysterectomy sometimes prescribed for endometriosis. If you do decide to wait it out, the following may prove helpful in the meantime.

✤ CHASTEBERRY is remarkably effective in the treatment of endometriosis.[6] It works through the pituitary, the "master gland" of the body. As mentioned below, under "Estrogen," it is also effective in promoting hormonal balance by regulating progesterone in relation to estrogen.

✤ EVENING PRIMROSE OIL or other sources of Omega-3 fatty acids, which reduce inflammation, may also be helpful. Experiment with the dose.

ENERGY

There are many natural energizers to choose from. The advantage to using them is they work with the body's resources, strengthening and soothing, rather than flogging an already weakened or exhausted system. Though some herbs or herbal combinations can provide you with almost an

---

6 Hobbs, Christopher, *Let's Live*, 12/88, p. 73.

instant "pick-me-up," even these are better for your body than singled-out, active ingredient drugs. EPHEDRA, for example, is gentler in its actions than pseudoephedrine, which is derived from EPHEDRA.

Just because something is a natural (i.e., nontampered-with) herb, however, does not mean it is automatically 100 percent safe. Natural substances, foods included, must be used with intelligence. EPHEDRA, for all its well-documented benefits, can raise blood pressure. For most people, this will not be a problem, for someone with high blood pressure already, another herb should be chosen. As I'm sure you've noticed, there are many herbs that are useful for any particular health problem and any given herb may be useful for many problems. Like Garrison Keillor's Powder Milk Biscuits, herbs can also be used to give you "the strength to get up and do what has to be done."

✸ ASTRAGALUS, enhances not only your immune system, but also your energy.

✸ AVENA, also known as OATS or OATMEAL, and even OATSTRAW, can nourish your nerves and your adrenal glands, thus providing you with sustained and sustainable energy. A cup of AVENA infusion at least once a week is rejuvenating in other ways, too, including for bones, nerves, skin, and hair.

✸ BEE POLLEN, though not strictly an herb, does come from herbs (via bees, of course). It gives energy, stamina, and good health. CAUTION: Some people are allergic to BEE POLLEN. Try a small amount under the tongue to see if you react before taking capsules.

✸ CAYENNE is a great daily tonic which will benefit the heart, circulation, and energy levels. Take about ¼ teaspoon in a glass of water or juice three times a day, or put it into capsules. It's also available already in capsules.

✸ DAMIANA, aphrodisiac and hormonal balancer, is also energizing.

✸ FO-TI aids the entire endocrine system, strengthening, rejuvenating, and energizing as a result. An excellent tonic.

✸ GARLIC, among all the wonders it performs, also strengthens and energizes the body. Those ancient Egyptian workers and Roman soldiers had it right, all along.

✸ GINGER is stimulating and, with frequent doses, will warm you up. Be aware that it is also an emmenagogue, and can promote bleeding.

❧ GOTU KOLA will give you stamina and energy. Combine it with CAYENNE and SIBERIAN GINSENG and you'll be a real powerhouse. It's also supposed to improve memory, prevent or allay senility, and promote longevity.

❧ KELP or other SEAWEED will prevent fatigue by nourishing your body and all your glands, including the thyroid and adrenals. Take one teaspoon of KELP granules or the equivalent of one gram (1000 mg.).

❧ NETTLE reduces fatigue by aiding adrenals and nourishing your entire body. Two cups of NETTLE infusion each day is a good dose. It even helps those with Epstein-Barr virus.

❧ PENNYROYAL is calming, yet energy-supporting. Don't take this herb if you are pregnant. It has been used to promote abortions.

❧ YERBA MATÉ has long been used for stamina and energy.

❧ SIBERIAN GINSENG, an adaptogen, is also justifiably famous for its stamina and energy producing properties. It is really good in combination with GOTU KOLA and CAYENNE.

❧ SARSAPARILLA is also good in combination with SIBERIAN GINSENG for energy and "get up and go."

❧ LICORICE ROOT, by aiding and abetting the adrenals, also energizes. It also helps to stabilize blood sugar levels, which will in turn aid in maintaining energy. A pinch of LICORICE ROOT POWDER, by the way, tastes sweet, not "licorishy," and makes a good sweetener for herbal teas. CAUTION: Don't take large doses of LICORICE ROOT if you have high blood pressure or hyperadrenal function.

❧ SCHIZANDRA is used by many groups around the world for energy. One group, a hunting tribe in northern China, called the Nanajas, often hunt all day without eating, after ingesting a few SCHIZANDRA berries. Ditto for hunters in eastern Siberia. It's said to have helped Russian pilots withstand lack of oxygen in the 1940s. It's also said to accelerate the body's "restorative processes." CAUTION. It should not be used by epileptics, people with high intracranial pressure, severe hypertension, or high acidity.

❧ EPHEDRA, also known as BRIGHAM TEA, DESERT TEA, MORMON TEA, and SQUAW TEA, is often used for sinus, bronchitis, asthma, and weight loss, but it is also energizing. CAUTION: It should not be used by anyone with high blood pressure or anyone who is really weak and debilitated, unless it's in an herbal combination in a small amount. Taken later in the day, it keeps some people awake.

ESTROGEN, HORMONAL BALANCE

Giving your hormones an "attitude adjustment" with herbs is a much gentler, kinder method than using synthetic estrogen. Herbs, for one thing, are complete, synergistic systems, designed to work as a whole, not as a single, possibly harmful, ingredient. Taking progesterone and estrogen at or after menopause produces a risk of breast cancer four times higher than for those who take no drugs at all. Taking only estrogen creates a risk that is twice that of the no-drugs group. As a whole, allopathic medicine downplays the cancer risk involved in estrogen replacement therapy (ERT or HRT, hormone replacement therapy), saying the benefits outweigh the risks, that cancer can be handled these days. The problem with that reasoning is that they don't mind lopping off or cutting out the "offending" parts, bombarding bodies with harsh chemicals or radiation (which sometimes produce more cancers), and taking immense amounts of your money and, possibly, your life. It's true that synthetic ERT can prevent or allay osteoporosis and other problems, but it is also true that other, safer methods can do so as well.

Hormonal balancing is a tricky thing, sometimes requiring trial and error dosage adjustments (those who take synthetic ERT go through this, too) before getting it right. This is not surprising if you consider how interconnected our bodily processes and ingredients are. Estrogen is not the only sex hormone necessary for the optimum function of our amazingly complex woman-system. A GOOD IDEA: Take liver strengthening herbs if you decide to do synthetic ERT. A good liver combination is: DANDELION ROOT, CELANDINE, BEET GREENS, OREGON GRAPE, and MILK THISTLE.

To further complicate matters, a particular herb or herbal combination may work just fine for a while and then seem to do no good whatsoever—even working well one day and seeming to turn off its benefits the next. The thing is, even during the apparently helter-skelter hormonal carchase known as menopause, there are cycles, variations in the hormonal mix coursing through your body and brain. These can be influenced even by the foods you eat. Solution: have several choices of herbs or combinations on hand and do kinetic testing, or, begin trusting your intuition more. You really do, at some level, know what is best for you. How will you get others to believe that if you don't?

✤ DONG QUAI, a Chinese herb which aids in estrogen replacement, or, more precisely, hormone balance, contains iron and vitamin E. Often dubbed the "female tonic." (See Herbal Notebook, "DONG QUAI—A WOMAN'S WONDER HERB.")

✤ BLACK COHOSH contains a natural precursor to estrogen (i.e., the body uses these elements as raw materials to produce its own hormones and only in the amount it needs), an antispasmodic, and emmenagogue. Native Americans used if for almost all "female complaints." Four capsules a day should be maximum dosage. CAUTION: Higher doses may cause vertigo and nerve center irritation, according to some sources; nausea and vomiting, according to others.

✤ BLESSED THISTLE, also an emmenagogue, among other things, is considered to be even more useful than BLACK COHOSH for hormonal imbalance.

✤ BURDOCK ROOT, said to be an aphrodisiac, containing estrogen precursors; a good tonic and healer.

✤ CHASTEBERRY, *Vitex, agnus-castus*, is a favorite herb in Europe, proclaimed to "work wonders" for all menopausal symptoms. The list of symptoms it can alleviate is truly exhaustive. Pharmacological studies have indicated it works mainly through the pituitary, our master gland, which regulates all other glands, including those that produce sexual hormones. Also of interest: CHASTEBERRY contains estrogen- and progesterone-like compounds.

✤ FO-TI, *Polygonum multiflorum*, is a tonic and nutritive herb for all the glands, especially the reproductive organs. It's also said to promote longevity and, in large doses, to be an aphrodisiac.

✤ DAMIANA, a reported aphrodisiac, is also a hormone balancer for both sexes. In addition, it is good for nerves and kidneys.

✤ SIBERIAN GINSENG, a well-known tonic and hormone balancer for both men and women, improves stamina and energy levels. Contains progesterone and testosterone precursors, as well as an anti-carcinogenic.

✤ KELP or other SEAWEED should be eaten or taken daily. You'll find it a great emotional roller-coaster-riding aid, plus helpful in alleviating or eliminating or preventing all menopausal symptoms.

✤ OATS, whether eaten or infused, will nourish and help balance your hormonal system. An infusion of OATSTRAW will do likewise.

℅ NETTLE leaves, either drunk as an infusion or eaten as a green vegetable, like SEAWEED, are superbly nourishing to the entire endocrine system. Among other things, they are a good source of calcium, magnesium, chlorophyll, chromium, plus many other minerals and vitamins. Two cups a day is often recommended. Another wonder herb for us wonder women!

℅ SARSAPARILLA, contains progesterone and testosterone hormone precursors. When combined with SIBERIAN GINSENG, SARSAPARILLA is said to promote energy and "ambition." This is very interesting, considering that menopausal women often report lethargy (no "ambition") and fatigue as symptoms. Though long known as a restorative for male reproductive organs, it benefits and energizes women, as well, especially during the latter half of the menstrual cycle when progesterone is in ascendancy over estrogen.

℅ LICORICE ROOT, a restorative and stimulant for the adrenal glands, in fact contains cortisone-like elements similar to the adrenal hormones. This is helpful in menopause because, as the ovaries begin to cease their hormone production, the adrenal glands step up their hormonal functions in an attempt to compensate for loss of estrogen. If the adrenals can't keep up, menopausal symptoms intensify. CAUTION: Use carefully or not at all (especially in substantial doses) if you have high blood pressure or are taking digitalis-based drugs. Be sure to get plentiful amounts of potassium if taking LICORICE ROOT.

℅ FALSE UNICORN ROOT is used for almost any uterine complaint, including hormonal imbalance, though it is generally combined with other herbs. Some report it is an aphrodisiac, as well.

℅ RED RASPBERRY leaf tea is a delicious drink and a wonderful tonic for the uterus and mucous membranes. It will also symptomatically allay cramping and almost any discomfort below the waist.

℅ SQUAW VINE, though used traditionally mainly for pregnancy and childbirth, is also an excellent uterine tonic and is helpful with congestion of the uterus and ovaries.

℅ SUMA is another herb containing estrogen precursors. It's also a rich source of germanium (gerMANium, not geRANium!), thought to enhance the flow of oxygen to cells. It's adaptagenic and tonic.

℅ ALFALFA, taken as tablets or tea, promotes estrogen production. ANISE SEED tea will too, as will SAGE tea and GARLIC.

🐚 ONIONS, DILL, and THYME reduce estrogen production.

🐚 EVENING PRIMROSE OIL aids in hormone balancing. Quite a bit of clinical research supports this. It contains precursors of prostaglandins, important to the proper functioning of every cell in your body. Some women report losing weight when they take 4 to 8 capsules of EVENING PRIMROSE OIL daily.

🐚 SAW PALMETTO BERRIES are a nutritive tonic for the reproductive organs of both men and women.

🐚 BLACK COHOSH, SARSAPARILLA ROOT, SIBERIAN GINSENG, LICORICE ROOT, FALSE UNICORN ROOT, BLESSED THISTLE and SQUAW VINE, combined in Nature's Way's Change-O-Life™, have aided many women through the menopause, nourishing the reproductive organs to make the event less stressful.

FIBROIDS

Fibroid growths (benign tumors made of fibrous material) can occur in the breasts, within the uterus, attached to the outside of it, or within the uterine wall. They can be small or can become quite large, exerting pressure on other organs. They can produce irregular periods, profuse bleeding, or pain.

The incidence of fibroids increases in the 40s and 50s, possibly aggravated by fluctuating hormone production. After menopause, though, they tend to shrink and even disappear. While waiting for that to happen, you may want to try any of the following treatments.

🐚 SEAWEED, such as KELP, eaten or taken daily, is useful for the prevention and healing of fibroids (cysts, too). About one teaspoon of KELP per day works well and quickly.

🐚 Many women have had success in eliminating infection, fibroids, or other growths in the uterus with a homemade herbal tampon. Says herbalist, H. Santillo, "[with this method] I have seen a fibroid tumor completely disappear in one month that was so large it blocked the colon and inhibited bowel movements."[7] Santillo's method: cut natural, undyed cotton cloth into 2- by 4-inch pieces. Make about a 1-inch pile, and with one end of a foot-long string, tie the middle of the pile. You should have about 10 inches of string left. Now mix equal amounts

---

7 Santillo, Humbart, *Natural Healing with Herbs*, Hohm Press, Arizona, 1984, p. 335.

of SLIPPERY ELM powder, WHITE OAK BARK powder, and enough water and FRENCH CLAY (or other powdered clay) to make a thin solution. Soak the tampon in the mixture until it is completely saturated. Then, before going to bed for the night, insert the tampon into the vagina, leaving the long end of the string hanging out. Wear a sanitary napkin to catch any leakage. Do this five nights a week. Remove the tampon each morning and douche with an infusion of GOLDENSEAL and MYRRH, to which you have added one teaspoon of pure APPLE CIDER VINEGAR.

✤ CHASTEBERRY, *Vitex agnus-castus*, a popular herb for all sorts of women's problems for thousands of years. One of its uses is to eliminate fibroids. It is used either as a tincture, in encapsulated powdered form, or as a tea.

✤ An effective poultice for cysts and fibroids is ordinary CABBAGE LEAF. Macerate some leaves and apply over the affected area. This "draws out" the fibroid.

✤ Another good poultice is made from PLANTAIN, COMFREY, and LOBELIA.

✤ Drinking two cups a day of an infusion of one ounce of RED CLOVER blossoms and one ounce of VIOLET leaves to a pint of boiling water is also effective.

✤ Other helpful herbs are BLACK COHOSH, ECHINACEA, GOLDEN-SEAL, PAU D'ARCO, and BLESSED THISTLE.

✤ A CASTOR OIL pack over the affected area also works for many. Soak a cloth in CASTOR OIL, place it over the area, cover with a sheet of plastic wrap or a plastic bag, cover the plastic with a heating pad, then cover all that with a towel or blanket. Keep this on for at least an hour. Do this several times a week, if not every night, until all is well again. It may take a month or more.

HAIR

Many people don't realize that wonderful hair depends on wonderful nourishment and kind care. The following herbs and oil treatments can help you give your hair what it needs during the menopause and beyond.

Herbs for Healthy Hair

❧ Take all, or one, or several of the following herbs over a period of time: HORSETAIL, NETTLE, PARSLEY, KELP, ONIONS, CAYENNE, ROSEMARY, RASPBERRY LEAF, SAGE, BURDOCK.

For Gray Hair

❧ Henna was used by ancient civilizations to dye hair, beards, horse's manes and tails, nails, palms of the hands and soles of the feet. It produces a reddish tint, or bright auburn hair color by itself. When mixed with Indigo, the result tends toward blue-black. Mixed half and half with CHAMOMILE, it yields a more reddish-brown color. Henna nourishes as well as colors the hair. It also protects it from the ravages of pollution and sun damage. It will gradually wash out in eight to twelve weeks. If you want to try it, you'd probably better test a strand or two first, before doing your whole head. Henna may turn gray or white hair various shades of bright orange! The color will vary according to the strength of the henna infusion.

❧ SAGE tea will darken graying hair. Steep about one-half cup of SAGE leaves in two cups of boiled water for several hours. Strain the liquid and pour it through your hair several times. Don't rinse. Towel off excess and let it dry.

❧ The same can be done with CHAMOMILE to bring out blond highlights.

For Dry, Falling Hair

❧ Dry, falling hair can be one of the side effects of birth-control pills.

❧ Two heaping tablespoons of SEA SALT mixed into a quart of boiling water, then cooled, is a simple remedy many have used. A little is rubbed into the scalp, daily, after shampooing.

❧ Pour boiling water over equal amounts of ROSEMARY and SAGE. Let steep five to fifteen minutes. Cool the liquid and massage into hair and scalp. Towel dry. Over time, this will improve your hair's condition; it is also likely to darken its color.

❧ If hair is dry and brittle, hot oil treatments are good. Here's one method: Warm two tablespoons of OLIVE OIL in a double boiler or similar set-up. When it's as hot as you can stand it, gently massage it into your scalp. Wrap a towel, wrung out in hot water, around your head for half an hour to an hour or so. Reheat the towel several times as it cools. Then wash your hair with a mild, herbal shampoo, using some APPLE CIDER VINEGAR as the last rinse. Hint for washing out oil: apply the shampoo and massage through your hair before adding water.

✻ Taking a tablespoon or two of WHEAT GERM OIL morning and evening will also be beneficial.

✻ It also helps to bend over, lowering your head, every time you shampoo, apply oil, or towel-dry your hair. Do it whenever you think of it throughout the day, too. This gets more life-bringing blood to your scalp.

✻ Prepare an herbal oil (See Herbal Notebook) using OLIVE OIL and NETTLE—the roots, leaves, or, if you can get it, the entire plant. Let it "mellow" for a month, then apply a warmed spoonful or so to your scalp at night, wash your hair in the morning. This is good to do once a week or so.

For Falling Hair

✻ KELP, in "ample supply" is said to prevent this.

✻ MARSHMALLOW leaf tea applied to the scalp will help prevent falling hair, as will ROSEMARY leaf tea, and a decoction of SAGE. So will NETTLE tea consumed daily and used as a rinse.

✻ PEACH LEAF tea, one cup consumed daily, will prevent or reverse falling hair.

For Hair Growth Stimulation

✻ CHASTEBERRY taken in capsule form or drunk as a daily tea has been used for hair growth.

✻ RED RASPBERRY LEAF tea or hair rinse will promote growth.

✻ Dr. Christopher's (Nature's Way's) BF & C™ Combination (WHITE OAK BARK, COMFREY LEAF, GRAVEL ROOT, MARSHMALLOW HERB, MULLEIN, BLACK WALNUT HULLS, SLIPPERY ELM, CAL-ENDULA, SKULLCAP), used as a fomentation, has been used for hair growth. Soak a natural, undyed, cotton cloth or stocking cap in a strong infusion of the BF&C combination. Place it on your head and cover with a shower cap, plastic wrap, or swimming cap, before retiring each night, for six weeks or so. This has also been known to clear stubborn scalp conditions.

✥ Dr. Christopher had another recipe for growing hair (even, he said, for the completely bald!). It's called the three-oil massage: Massage head with CASTOR OIL, in a clockwise circular motion, once a day for two days. The next two days, use OLIVE OIL, followed by WHEAT GERM OIL for two more days. On the seventh day, give your head a rest. Right after each massage, Dr. Christopher recommended sitting with your head uncovered in the sun, beginning with two minutes and working up to a maximum of 30 minutes. This should be done in direct sunlight, but not during the hottest part of the day. If it's cloudy, use a sunlamp. You then wash your hair with a mild, natural shampoo. Keep this up as long as necessary.

✥ Another treatment said to promote hair growth uses BURDOCK seed oil. Pour some into your palm and rub it into your scalp. Cover your head with a hot, wet towel for an hour or more, then shampoo. Repeat weekly as needed. It's also helpful to drink BURDOCK leaf or BURDOCK seed tea along with this treatment.

✥ Here's another method to stimulate hair growth, even for hair loss due to chemotherapy: Make a decoction of NETTLE root and rub your scalp every morning and night with it. Or do the same with from 5–90 drops of tincture in water. Drinking from one-half to one cup of NETTLE root infusion a day along with the treatment will also help, or, if you're not into tea drinking, eat the cooked seed or leaves of NETTLE daily.

✥ One part ROSEMARY OIL to 2 parts JOJOBA OIL in 8 parts water (purified, if possible), shaken vigorously before applying, is also effective for stimulating hair growth. If hair follicles are still alive, even the completely bald may be surprised at the results.

✥ PEACH LEAF tea, one cup consumed daily, is said to promote hair growth.

For Thick, Lustrous, Glossy Hair

✥ Grind 35–40 BURDOCK seeds and steep in a cup of boiling water. You may take half a cupful up to six times a day. Or take 20 to 40 drops of BURDOCK seed tincture in water two or three times a day.

♚ Another route to gorgeous hair: eat half a cup of cooked NETTLE greens several days a week or drink a cup of NETTLE tea every day, or at least three or four times a week. Also, use this NETTLE tea hair rinse once a week: Pour one pint of boiling water over half an ounce of dried NETTLE leaves, cover, and let set overnight. Next day, strain and, if you wish, add one tablespoon of NETTLE root tincture to the liquid. Or, make some NETTLE vinegar (see Herbal Notebook), add a tablespoon to a cup of water, and use as a hair rinse once a week.

♚ RASPBERRY LEAF, drunk as a tea or used as a rinse, promotes thick, beautiful hair.

♚ Take or eat SEAWEED, such as KELP or DULSE, every day.

HEADACHES, MIGRAINE, OR OTHER

♚ If you haven't always had migraine headaches, hormonal imbalance could be the villain. If you suspect this to be the cause, try the herbs under "Estrogen," above, such as SIBERIAN GINSENG and SARSA-PARILLA. That may do the trick for you, or, try any of the following.

♚ GINGER, fresh or powdered, has been used to successfully treat and prevent migraine headaches. Powdered GINGER, 500–600 mg. (about one capsule's worth), is taken with a glass of water as soon as the "aura" which often signals the beginning of a migraine is noticed. Two capsules are then taken once every four hours for four or five days. Continued daily use of GINGER, either in capsule form or fresh, as part of the diet, is said to prevent or greatly reduce migraine occurrence.[8]

♚ ROSEMARY infusion, steeped for 5 to 15 minutes, and taken in doses of two ounces at a time, three times daily will also help migraines. Or, make ROSEMARY oil and take one-half to 3 drops a day in warm water or tea. CAUTION: ROSEMARY can raise blood pressure. Do not exceed three cups of ROSEMARY tea a day.

♚ FENUGREEK seed tea, made by steeping them for 5 to 15 minutes, is also used for migraines. A cup or two a day is usually recommended.

♚ FEVERFEW is another herb reported to prevent migraine attacks. CAUTION: A small percentage of those taking FEVERFEW reported the side effect of sores in the mouth. Taking vitamin C eliminated this problem.

---

8 Mustafa, T. and Brivastava, K. D., *Journal of Ethnopharmacology*, 29(1990) 267-278; *Herbal Health-line*, Vol. 2, No. 1, p. 15.

✽ The Change-O-Life™ formula mentioned under "Estrogen," as well as any of the other herbs in that section, have also been known to alleviate headaches, especially if they appear to be connected to hot flashes or hormone imbalance.

✽ WOOD BETONY is good for a tension headache.

HEART PALPITATIONS

WARNING: Do not suddenly stop taking a prescription drug for your heart without consulting a physician—preferably a nutritionally-oriented one. Palpitations occur in about 48 percent of menopausal women. A distressing symptom, it can nevertheless be handled by any of several different herbs.

✽ MOTHERWORT is a specific in cases of palpitations induced by endocrine (glandular) or functional nervous disorders. Use the fresh herb if you can, or obtain the freshest of dried MOTHERWORT that you can. It loses strength rapidly in storage. Make an infusion and drink a cup or so daily. It is an excellent cardiac tonic in general.

✽ HAWTHORN BERRIES are also excellent for palpitations and for use as a cardiac tonic. (It is also used for cardiac edema, arrhythmia, arteriosclerosis, high blood pressure, and just plain strengthening of the heart.) Hawthorn is often used as a tincture, syrup, or extract. Start with a couple of drops four times a day, working up to ten drops four times a day. Do this for two weeks, stop for a day or two, then start up again. CAUTION: Unless you are absolutely certain you know the plant, do not pick your own berries to prepare. Hawthorn is sometimes called "THORN APPLE," and could be confused with a poisonous member of the NIGHTSHADE family (*Solanaceae*) which is also called "THORN APPLE."

✽ GINGER diminishes thromboxane production, and this, in turn, reduces the risk of heart attacks and strokes from blood clots.

HOT FLASHES AND NIGHT SWEATS

Hot flashes are the result of vasomotor instability, to use the medical term. The vasomotor nerves are the body's thermostat-controllers. It's their job to regulate body temperature by controlling the diameter of the blood vessels. A disturbance in hormone levels interferes with the signals transmitted to the vasomotor nerves, and hot flashes, dizziness, and sometimes heart palpitations, result. As your system finally adjusts to the lower or different levels of hormones, the symptoms will abate. There is help in the meantime, though.

❧ DAMIANA, DONG QUAI, CHASTEBERRY, BLACK COHOSH, and other herbs listed under "Estrogen," above, including the Change-O-Life™ formula, have all been used successfully to stop these annoying symptoms. Some women find they need to take up to two capsules three times a day, perhaps for two weeks, before symptoms are eliminated.

INSOMNIA

❧ CATNIP tea will calm you down (unless you're a cat), let you relax and go to sleep. Take a cupful two to three times throughout the day and just before bedtime; or just before bedtime may be all you need.

❧ The same can be said for CHAMOMILE tea. It's extremely soothing and also delicious.

❧ SKULLCAP, HOPS FLOWERS, VALERIAN, BLUE VERVAIN, MOTHERWORT, YARROW, BASIL, VIOLET LEAVES, and LADY SLIPPER are all relaxing and calming, whether you take them in capsules or as a tea. Use one of these herbs or any combination of them.

❧ A decoction of CELERY SEED or root is another good choice. Have a cupful half an hour or so before retiring.

❧ A formula by Dr. Christopher, called Silent Night™ by Nature's Way, combines HOPS FLOWERS, VALERIAN ROOT, and SKULLCAP. The suggested dose is two to six capsules before bed; or, in really tough cases, two capsules 4 to 6 hours before bedtime and then two to six capsules at bedtime.

❧ The combination for calcium, under "Depression" will also help: COMFREY, ALFALFA, OATSTRAW, HORSETAIL, IRISH MOSS.

❧ PASSION FLOWER is another good choice against insomnia.

❧ CHASTEBERRY, that ever-useful herb, will also put insomnia to rout.

❧ Have a cup of any of the above herbal teas for insomnia, and take a nap. Oddly enough, many people sleep better at night if they take a nap in the afternoon.

INVOLUNTARY, FREQUENT, OR BURNING URINATION

Decreasing estrogen thins the lining of the bladder, as well as of the vagina. The bladder lining is then more susceptible to irritations and infections. This can result in involuntary urination (especially upon sneezing, coughing, or vigorous laughing), an urgent need to urinate frequently, or a sensation of burning upon urination. Estrogen-providing herbs and foods can help to relieve these symptoms, as can one or more of the following herbal treatments.

❧ AGRIMONY, taken as a strong tea, between 4 and 6 P.M.

❧ YARROW tea may also be used in the same manner as AGRIMONY, and SHEPHERD'S PURSE has also been found useful.

❧ A decoction of CELERY root or seeds is also good for incontinence. Interestingly enough, it is also good for urine retention and dropsy (edema).

❧ MARSHMALLOW root is a good choice to use in conjunction with other herbs. Use ½ to 1 teaspoon of the tincture three times a day, or take 5 to 10 of #0 capsules three times a day, or make a decoction and drink 6 ounces three times a day. (See Herbal Notebook.)

❧ A tincture of PLANTAIN is also helpful. An infusion made of the leaves has also been found useful. Drink half a cup, two or three times a day.

❧ BUCHU, CORN SILK, FENNEL SEED, and WOOD BETONY, taken individually or combined, as an infusion are other herbs long used to soothe and heal the bladder and kidneys.

❧ The following combination will help to tone and strengthen the kidneys: 1 part PLANTAIN, 1 part SLIPPERY ELM, 2 parts GOLDENSEAL, 1 part UVA URSI, ½ part GINGER. Combine and prepare an infusion, drinking half a cup every few hours.

❧ KELP, which contains many nutrients, including potassium, strengthens the urinary tract.

❧ OREGON GRAPE ROOT, as a tincture, decoction, extract, or capsules, is beneficial for the kidneys. It also has antiseptic qualities.

MEMORY

✍ BLESSED THISTLE reportedly gets more oxygen to the brain, thereby "revving" it up and improving memory.

✍ GINKGO also has the reputation of stimulating the memory and has even been credited with helping Alzheimer's patients in the early stages. Studies indicate GINKGO improves the oxygen supply to the brain and does enhance mental efficiency. It improves circulation in general. A rich source of antioxidants and bioflavonoids, it reportedly healed one person[9] of macular degeneration. It is taken in capsules or as an extract.

✍ BAYBERRY is another herb that is beneficial for the brain.

✍ The ever-useful KELP is—guess what?—also brain food. Try to get some every day.

✍ GOTU KOLA, YERBA MATÉ, SIBERIAN GINSENG, and PASSION FLOWER also have a long history of reported memory and concentration improvement.

MENSTRUATION

Menstruation doesn't just magically stop one day when you reach a certain age. It's a bit like puberty in reverse. As menopause approaches, there can be irregular periods, erratic and delayed periods, extra heavy or light periods, and sometimes painful periods, even if menstruation has been going like clockwork for you for years. Irregular periods can be expected before and sometimes with menopause. This can occur every so often at any age, perhaps related to stress or diet or intense exercise.

Between-period bleeding is usually not serious, but it can be. If it happens after age 40, after skipping periods, it's likely to be just a signal that menopause is beginning to "think about" occurring. If between-period bleeding occurs only after sex, it could be a minor or a serious cervical problem. See a doctor to get a diagnosis. Then you decide on the treatment you prefer.

✍ Any of the herbs mentioned under "Estrogen" will be helpful for regulating periods. CHASTEBERRY would be a good choice.

---

9 *Better Nutrition*, 12/92, p. 8, letter from reader.

❧ DONG QUAI is helpful in regulating menses—and starting them—but it should not be taken if there is excessive menstrual flow.

❧ ANGELICA, *Angelica archangelica*, could be used instead of DONG QUAI to start delayed menstruation, but its action is somewhat harsher.

❧ CRAMPBARK, STRAWBERRY LEAF, and WILD YAM will all ease heavy, painful periods.

❧ SQUAW VINE is also used for menstrual irregularities. A good herbal combination with it is: 1 part SQUAW VINE, 2 parts RASPBERRY LEAVES, 1 part BLUE COHOSH, 1 part BLACK COHOSH, 1 part FALSE UNICORN. Mix and prepare an infusion, taking a cup or two a day, or powder the herbs and place in capsules.

❧ BLUE COHOSH root is taken for cramps and to start or regulate menses. It should not be taken if pregnant, unless you want to induce delivery. (It's said to promote a painless and rapid delivery.)

❧ FALSE UNICORN has long been used for uterine disorders, cramps, and to prevent miscarriage.

❧ OATS, taken daily as food, as an infusion, or as a tincture, are excellent for ovarian and uterine disorders. The tincture should be made from fresh OATS (the grain, called "groats," not the rolled "OATMEAL" familiar as a breakfast cereal) which have been harvested when the milky substance is present in the grain. Thirty to sixty drops are taken three times a day.

❧ BLACK COHOSH is also used for menstrual pain, either ovarian or uterine, and for regulation.

❧ SKULLCAP is also used for pains of ovarian or uterine origin.

❧ RED RASPBERRY LEAF tea will soothe the savage cramp and help to control frequent or excessive bleeding. It will tone the uterus, as well.

❧ For heavy periods, NETTLE tea will also slow the flow.

❧ MYRRH gum will encourage delayed menses to get with it and will also allay menstrual pain. Two to six #0 capsules, or 30 to 60 drops of tincture, or 3 oz. of infusion, three times a day is a common dosage. CAUTION: MYRRH should not be taken over a long period of time or in large amounts. In sizable amounts it can be toxic.

OSTEOPOROSIS

The word means, literally, porosity of the bones, and that's exactly what happens when not enough calcium is deposited to keep up with accelerated bone loss as estrogen production decreases. Estrogen is important in the manufacture of new bone tissue, and when it becomes scarce, bones become riddled with holes or "air pockets," like Swiss cheese or sponges. They become brittle and easily broken. Roughly 200,000 women a year are disabled by hip fractures and resulting falls. The weakened bone can no longer take the weight of the body, the hip breaks, and the woman falls. Many die each year due to complications from these injuries or the resulting surgeries. Others lose height (and gain pain) from collapsing vertebrae and/or develop the infamous "dowager's hump."

This estrogen dip and accelerated calcium loss occurs long before the last period. The calcium loss can continue for as long as ten years afterward. Postmenopausal women need even more calcium than youngsters require at puberty.[10] Fortunately, you can do something about this: avoid fluoridated water (which actually extracts calcium from the bones), eat less, or no, red meat (too much phosphorus, it requires more calcium in the blood stream—often taken from bones—to balance it), ditto for soft drinks, don't smoke, eat calcium-rich[11] and boron-rich[12] foods, exercise, avoid excess caffeine and alcohol, take calcium and magnesium supplements and some of the following herbs. Herbs previously listed under "Estrogen," above, will also be helpful.

✤ HORSETAIL, also known as SHAVEGRASS, contains silicon in an easily absorbable form. This improves calcium utilization, strengthens bones, and is important in collagen production. Collagen is part of what "holds us altogether."

✤ ALFALFA is a magnificent source of minerals, vitamins, and chlorophyll. Use as a tea or take tablets and more tablets and more tablets. Chew them like candy if you get tired of swallowing them! They taste good, sort of green and grassy.

---

10 Weiner, Michael, Ph.D., *Herbal Healthline*, Vol. 2, No. 1, 1991.

11 For example: yogurt, milk, cheese, sunflower seeds, sesame seeds, corn tortillas, oats, soybeans and tofu, kale, broccoli, mustard, dandelion, and collard greens. Try rolling a banana in sesame seeds as part of breakfast or for a snack.

12 For example: nuts, apples, pears, grapes, leafy vegetables, plus there is a little in whole grains, but only a trace in dairy products, fish, or red meats. Boron, in the amount of 3 mg. a day, greatly enhances calcium utilization.

✿ DANDELION leaves, eaten as cooked greens or added to salads, or taken in capsules or as tea, are a source of calcium and magnesium, plus other vitamins and minerals. (Calcium and magnesium are synergistic cousins; each helps the other.)

✿ OATS and OATSTRAW are also good sources of calcium.

✿ KELP, or other SEAWEED, eaten or taken daily, is another fine source of many vitamins and minerals, including calcium. It does so many things for us, it's a wonder the women of the world aren't flocking to the seashores to graze.

✿ Here's a formula for a mineral syrup good for hair and nails, as well as bones. Combine equal amounts of the following to make four ounces and add to one quart of water: PARSLEY ROOT AND LEAF, YELLOW DOCK, NETTLE LEAF, HORSETAIL, COMFREY ROOT, IRISH MOSS, KELP, WATERCRESS. Simmer gently until the liquid is reduced by half. Strain off the liquid and reserve. Cover the herbs with water again and simmer for ten minutes. Strain and simmer the combined decoctions until the volume is again reduced by half. Add an equal amount of blackstrap molasses. Keep refrigerated and take one tablespoonful several times a day.

✿ Dr. Christopher's BF & C™ formula is almost a "magic" aid to bone and cartilage building. Two capsules taken three times a day is the usual dose.

✿ BONESET leaf tea (about one teaspoon to one cup of boiling water)—drinking several cupfuls per day will relieve aching bone pain.

✿ Here's an interesting VINEGAR tincture for calcium: Collect eggshells from one dozen eggs,[13] dry them, and remove the membranes. Powder the shells, using a blender or mortar and pestle, and add to a pint of pure APPLE CIDER VINEGAR. This will bubble and fizz wonderfully, so use a quart or larger glass jar or bottle and call in the grandkids to watch. Immediately cap the jar. Take a tablespoon three times a day.

---

13 From non-commercial (hence, non-chemicalized) sources, if possible. Vinegar has antiseptic properties, but eggshells can also be heated during the drying process, to eliminate any harmful bacteria.

SEX

About 20 percent of menopausal women experience decreased sex drive. (Good news! That means 80 percent do not!) Some women report an increased sex drive, and the remainder evidently continue as they always were. Whatever your case, you may at some time find occasion to use one or more of the following herbs, some reported (with some authority) to be aphrodisiacs. Henry Kissinger's famous quote to the contrary (that "power is the best aphrodisiac"), positive health and attitudes are the best aphrodisiacs of all. Maintaining or improving your hormonal balance (see "Estrogen" section, above) will solve a lot of problems, too.

❧ OATS (or AVENA), believe it or not, can enhance your sex life! Because of the ability to aid in nervous disorders, oats have been used in tincture form, 30 to 60 drops three times a day, for sexual neurasthenia (no feeling "down there"). OATS are also nutritive and rejuvenating for the endocrine system and will improve health in general. OATS will enrich your sexual pleasure because they nurture your nerves; caressing and being caressed will become a joy again. Have a cup of OAT infusion at least once a week and eat OATMEAL often.

❧ DAMIANA enjoys a long-time reputation as an aphrodisiac and energy-enhancer for both men and women.

❧ SAW PALMETTO is a reproductive system nutritive tonic for women and men (especially helpful for a man if he has an enlarged prostate), a sexual stimulant, and, as a tincture combined with tincture of OATS, is also useful in the treatment of sexual neurasthenia.

❧ FALSE UNICORN is another aphrodisiac of long-standing repute.

❧ FENUGREEK decoction is also considered an aphrodisiac.

❧ FO-TI is said to be a rejuvenator of the endocrine glands and, hence, an effective tonic and nutritive herb. In large doses, it acts as an aphrodisiac.

❧ GOTU KOLA, known in India as the longevity herb, is also a rejuvenator, similar in effect to FO-TI.

❧ SIBERIAN GINSENG and SARSAPARILLA will spark a sagging sex drive for both men and women. One herbalist reports that some female clients are wont to slip this combination into their husbands' food!

❧ SKULLCAP will subdue an excessive sex drive, especially combined with PENNYROYAL and CRAMPBARK and/or with HOPS.

SKIN

Are the words "age" spots, dry skin, and wrinkles suddenly finding their way into your vocabulary, pervading your thoughts, and jumping out at you from slick magazines? Don't despair! Once again, Mother Nature comes to your rescue. For lovely skin, you must first cleanse your body of toxins and then nourish it with unadulterated nutrients. Herbs can handle these jobs like rain runs down a rose petal—naturally and easily. But first, the simplest thing you can do for your health and for your skin is to drink plenty of good, pure water every day. Smiling a lot helps, too.

🎋 OATS or OATSTRAW infusion, drunk or bathed in, is extremely sooth-ing and nourishing to your skin. Here's an oldtime recipe that makes your skin smooth and feels wonderful: Tie some OATMEAL in a small square of cotton or, to use a modern method, tie some in a knee-high hose and get into a warm or hot bath with it. Squeeze the OATS a bit until a milky cream exudes and use the bag of OATS as a scrub for your face and body. Your skin will feel silky and wonderful. This is good for itching, too, including from poison oak or poison ivy, even chicken pox.

🎋 An OATMEAL pack will work wonders for your face, soothing, smoothing, and nourishing it. Mix some ground OATMEAL with but-termilk or egg white to make a paste. You can grind the OATMEAL using your blender or food processor. Apply the paste to your face, leave it on 20 minutes or so, then rinse it off with cool water. If you fol-low this with a facial steam (see below) from an infusion of NETTLE, you'll be extremely pleased with the results.

🎋 For age spots, or liver spots, apply the juice that oozes from the stem of fresh DANDELION or from the cut or broken root. The root is favored for this treatment, but the stem juice works, too. This is one of those treatments that must be faithfully applied for some time.

🎋 Another treatment for age spots or other blotches is to drink, daily, a strong decoction of the root and leaves of AGRIMONY, (*Agrimonia eupatoria*).

🎋 The main treatment for these harmless, yet annoying to some people, age spots is to purify the blood. Herbalist Humbart Santillo[14] suggests the following formula: 1 part BARBERRY ROOT, 1 part WILD YAM, 1 part DANDELION, ½ part LICORICE ROOT. Simmer one ounce in

---

14 Santillo, Humbart, B. S., M. H., *Natural Healing with Herbs,* Hohm Press, Prescott, Arizona, 1991.

pint of water for ten minutes, then strain. Drink two ounces three to four times daily.

&⁊ The following herbs, mixed or taken separately, are also useful for age spots: DANDELION, RED CLOVER, PARSLEY ROOT, GOLD-ENSEAL, and BURDOCK ROOT.

&⁊ THISILYN, a MILK THISTLE seed extract (should contain at least 80 per cent silymarin) is also a potent liver detoxifier and protector, and therefore should be useful for age spots.

Remember, all these treatments for "spots" may take some months.

&⁊ A good blood purifying combination for skin, including for acne and other eruptions, is: 2 parts ECHINACEA, 1 part RED CLOVER, 1 part KELP, 1 part BURDOCK, 1 part DANDELION ROOT, 1 part SARSA-PARILLA, 1 part YELLOW DOCK, 1/2 part LICORICE ROOT, ⅛ part CAYENNE. Make a powder from the mixture with a blender or mortar and pestle, fill #00 capsules, and take two every two or three hours until the condition improves.

&⁊ A SASSAFRAS, SARSAPARILLA, and DANDELION decoction is good for skin, too. One cup three times a day.

&⁊ NETTLE tincture, 10-15 drops, four times a day is good for skin eruptions, as well. Also, wash your skin with NETTLE leaf infusion two or three times a day. NETTLE is wonderful for all kinds of skin and skin problems, including acne and eczema. For smooth, clear skin and healthy nails, drink NETTLE tea every day or eat half a cup of cooked NETTLE several times a week.

&⁊ A weekly steam facial using NETTLE, followed by applying the warm NETTLE leaves as a poultice or fomentation will eliminate blemishes and deter sun damage and loss of skin elasticity.

&⁊ Drinking infusions of DANDELION ROOT, PLANTAIN, ALFALFA, CHICKWEED, and/or PARSLEY, two to four cups per day, will produce healthy skin.

&⁊ KELP or other SEAWEED in capsule or granular form is also beneficial to your skin. Try a teaspoon of KELP a day in grapefruit or other juice.

&⁊ A steam facial, a method that moisturizes, cleans, and nourishes (by increasing blood flow to the surface of your face), can be enhanced by the use of herbs. Steam facials can help dry skin, dull, lifeless-looking skin, and clogged pores. Any of the following herbs may be used, alone or in combination. Some are aromatic, some are astringent. Here's how: Add a tablespoon or two of the dried herb or herbs to a quart of boiling water. Hold your face about a foot over the pan or bowl and cover your head with a towel, letting it form a tent over the container. Do this for five or ten minutes, then pat face dry with a clean towel and apply a moisturizer to hold in the moisture your skin has just absorbed. Some herbs for a steam facial: SAGE, YARROW, LAVENDER, PARSLEY, fresh or dried; FENNEL seeds, crushed, PEPPERMINT, SPEAR-MINT, EUCALYPTUS, THYME, WINTERGREEN, CHAMOMILE, ELDERBERRY flowers, or powdered LICORICE ROOT. A steam facial using crushed BURDOCK SEEDS is especially good for eliminating blackheads and whiteheads.

❧ To remove dried, flaky skin, try PAPAYA! Use one wedge or large slice of ripe PAPAYA. Remove the seeds, mash the pulp, then spread it over your face or wherever you need it. Leave it on only a couple of minutes, or it may be too drying. Wipe it off with a damp cloth and splash your skin with cool water.

❧ Another dead skin remover is a paste of LEMON juice and salt rubbed over the elbows, feet, or wherever needed.

❧ For dry, chapped hands make a MARIGOLD (also known as CALENDULA) infusion, or MARIGOLD petal ointment. (See Herbal Notebook.) A MARIGOLD infusion in the bath is reputed to reduce scars, soothe varicose veins, and help thread veins on the face.

❧ To prevent or eliminate wrinkles, don't smoke, drink plenty of water, get enough sleep, and use any of the following:

❧ Because silicon is important in the production of collagen, KELP and HORSETAIL, both high in silicon, are helpful for the prevention of wrinkling and sagging. These herbs feed your skin with many other nutrients, as well.

❧ Potassium is also an important ally against wrinkles. Some herbs high in potassium are: BLACK WALNUT HULLS, KELP, DULSE, HORSETAIL, WATERCRESS, SAGE, and ROSEMARY.

❧ A salve or ointment made with CHAMOMILE FLOWERS or extract will make wrinkles disappear like magic. Apply daily. You should notice a difference in three to seven days.

ஜ An infusion made from crushed BURDOCK SEEDS, half a cup several times a day, is another skin smoother. Twenty to forty drops of BUR-DOCK SEED tincture, taken four times a day in water, works well, too.

ஜ Smooth skin is another of NETTLE tea's wonder-working properties.

ஜ A lotion made from ELDERBERRY flowers is soothing and smoothing for your skin. (It's also good for just about any skin ailment.) To make it, pour one quart of boiling water over about a tablespoonful of dried ELDERBERRY flowers. Cover and let steep an hour. Then strain and apply the liquid to your skin, as a wash or fomentation.

ஜ ELDERBERRY leaf ointment, is also soothing, softening, and healing. (It can also be used for tumors, swelling, or wounds.) Prepare an ointment (See Herbal Notebook) using the following: 8 oz. ELDERBERRY leaves, 4 oz. PLANTAIN leaves, 2 oz. GROUND IVY (*Glechoma hederacea*), 4 oz. WORMWOOD.

VAGINAL DRYNESS

One symptom of the reduction of estrogen levels for some menopausal women is vaginal dryness, resulting in uncomfortable, if not painful, intercourse. All the herbs listed earlier, under "Estrogen," can help this problem. A salve or herbal oil made with WHEAT GERM OIL or VITAMIN E OIL, perhaps combined with ELDERBERRY FLOWERS, CALENDULA (MARIGOLD), CHAMOMILE, MARSHMALLOW, or SLIPPERY ELM BARK would be a good choice for a vaginal lubricant or suppository. Many say that VITAMIN E, suppositories or oil, works as well as estrogen cream. WHEAT GERM OIL, by the way, is a good source of VITAMIN E.

VAGINITIS, LEUKORRHEA, YEAST INFECTIONS

The walls of the vagina tend to thin as estrogen production falls off, and this can lead to vaginitis. Vaginitis is a rather inclusive term which describes several conditions or causes of irritation and inflammation of the vagina, usually with a discharge, odor, itching, and, sometimes, painful intercourse.

Vaginitis can be due to trichomoniasis (a protozoa), characterized by burning, itching, a thin, frothy discharge, and a rash. Hemophilus is non-specific vaginitis which produces a creamy white, yellowish or grayish discharge, sometimes bloody, accompanied by lower back pain, cramps, and swollen glands in both the abdomen and inner thighs. Leukorrhea, another type of vaginitis, produces a white, watery discharge and may be caused either by yeast infections or trichomonads.

Vaginitis can also be caused by yeast infections, sometimes called thrush or monilia, which exhibit curdy, profuse, odoriferous discharge, itching, and inflammation. Yeast infections are not really a yeast or an infection, but a yeast-like fungus, known as *Candida albicans.* The condition is actually known as candidiasis. One of the most common contributing factors to candidiasis is the modern ubiquitous usage of antibiotics, both by the medical profession and the meat industry. Along with the "bad" bacteria, antibiotics also kill off the "good" bacteria that we normally harbor. These good bacteria aid our digestion (ever notice gas problems after a round of antibiotics?), produce certain vitamins, and help keep many harmful organisms at bay. These harmful organisms include *Candida albicans,* which is always hanging around, waiting for the right conditions to proliferate. Stress, diabetes, whether diagnosed or not, and overindulgence in sugar are some other factors related to the "outbreak" of candidiasis.

For Yeast Infections

Douche with any, or a combination of, the following:

❧ GOLDENSEAL and MYRRH (combined), BAYBERRY BARK, BLACK WALNUT, COMFREY, SAGE, or YARROW. Recline in a tub for douching and hold the liquid in for several minutes by elevating the pelvis slightly or by holding the vagina opening closed with your hand. In addition to douching, taking these herbs internally as a tea or capsules would also be a good idea.

❧ OATSTRAW infusion is also good. Douche with it once a week and drink a cup or more of it daily for a month or so.

❧ PAU D'ARCO, ingested as capsules or tincture or used in a strong infusion as a douche, would be extremely helpful in "yeast" infections. It is famous for its antifungal properties. Take two capsules every three hours or as an infusion several times a day.

For Leukorrhea

❧ The following herbs are useful for douches: BAYBERRY, BLUE COHOSH, BLUE FLAG, LAVENDER, PAU D'ARCO, RED SAGE, SLIPPERY ELM, or WHITE OAK BARK. You can also make a suppository of powdered SLIPPERY ELM and a little water, adding one or more of the other powdered herbs if you wish.

For All Types of Vaginitis:

🍂 MYRRH combined with GOLDENSEAL in #00 capsules, should be taken two at a time every two hours.

🍂 MYRRH, alone, will also aid vaginitis. Take it as a tincture, extract, infusion, decoction, or in capsules. It may also be used as a douche. Use the same dosages as for OREGON GRAPE ROOT, below. CAUTION: MYRRH should not be taken for long periods of time or in large doses. It can be toxic.

🍂 For another good douche for vaginal discharges, prepare a strong infusion (1 ounce of herb to 1 pint of water) of equal parts of the following: GOLDENSEAL, RED RASPBERRY LEAF, ECHINACEA, SQUAW VINE, and SLIPPERY ELM. Strain and add one teaspoon of APPLE CIDER VINEGAR. Douche in the morning and try to hold for 5 minutes. It helps to recline in the tub to do this.

🍂 YELLOW DOCK may also be used as a douche, as above.

🍂 WHITE OAK BARK infusion is also used in this manner.

🍂 YARROW tincture, 5 to 20 drops, drunk three or four times a day in water, is also recommended.

🍂 UVA URSI may be used as a douche or taken as a tincture or infusion. For the infusion, steep UVA URSI for 30 minutes and take three ounces several times a day, up to three cups. The tincture is usually taken in 10 to 20 drop doses in water, three or four times a day.

🍂 OREGON GRAPE ROOT may be taken as a tincture at the rate of 30 to 60 drops, three times a day, or prepared as an infusion for a douche. (This herb will also aid your liver, kidneys, stomach, gall bladder, and thyroid, thereby improving all manner of conditions, including skin problems and constipation.)

🍂 APPLE CIDER VINEGAR douches (two tablespoons to a pint of warm water, twice a day a first, then once a day) are very effective. Even though yeast flourishes in an acidic environment, there is something in vinegar that inhibits its growth. Vinegar can also inhibit the growth of bacteria and trichomonads by establishing the proper acidity (pH) for the proliferation of "good" bacteria.

🍂 By crushing a clove of GARLIC in the vinegar solution and letting it sit a while before straining out the garlic and douching, you hit bacteria with a double whammy. Garlic is well-known for its antibiotic properties.

VARICOSE VEINS

Venous, or "used," blood from the feet and legs must be pumped back to the heart and lungs against gravity. There are valves in these veins which prevent the blood from flowing back to your feet. Varicose veins occur when these valves break down or malfunction. If one valve goes, extra pressure is exerted on the ones below it, and, if nothing is done, they, too, will eventually "blow." With the blood thus "pooling" in them, the veins expand and bulge. This is not only unsightly, but can also be painful. The condition can be the result of constipation ("straining"), liver malfunction, lack of exercise, or vitamin E deficiency. It's interesting to note that this condition is unknown in so-called "primitive" societies where they eat a fiber-rich, unprocessed diet (eliminates constipation) and are physically active.

❧ Liver purifying herbs and herbal combinations are good to take along with any other treatment for varicose veins. DANDELION, THISILYN, and OREGON GRAPE ROOT are good choices for single herbs. Nature's Way combinations Liveron™, Red Clover Combination™, and the combination listed under "Arthritis" would also be effective. Take as capsules or drink as teas.

❧ Herbs to aid the circulation would also be useful: BUTCHER'S BROOM, CAYENNE, GINGER, or PRICKLY ASH BARK fall into this category.

❧ Other herbs good for varicose veins: HORSE CHESTNUT, PAU D'ARCO, WHITE OAK BARK, MARSHMALLOW, MULLEIN, OATSTRAW, and BLACK WALNUT, taken as teas or tinctures in water.

❧ If edema is a problem, YARROW, PARSLEY, CORN SILK, or DANDELION teas will help.

❧ Poultices applied warm or hot that will help include: BAYBERRY, BLACK WALNUT, CALENDULA, WITCH HAZEL, TANSY, MULLEIN, WHITE OAK BARK, SAGE, OATSTRAW, SASSAFRAS, MARSHMALLOW, or WOOD SORREL.

❧ For ulcers on the legs, use poultices of COMFREY, SLIPPERY ELM, GOLDENSEAL, or CALENDULA. Or bathe the legs in a warm infusion of these herbs. Taking GOLDENSEAL, ECHINACEA, CHAPARRAL,[15] or PAU D'ARCO will help heal skin ulcers, too.

---

15 See Footnote 1, p. 5, for FDA ruling on this herb.

✇ HORSETAIL will also be helpful, supplying many minerals needed for proper functioning in all areas, as will ALFALFA, as will KELP.

✇ A bath or fomentation of an infusion of CALENDULA (MARIGOLD) or an ointment made from MARIGOLD petals will aid in reducing scars and will be soothing.

VOICE LOWERING

✇ CHASTEBERRY is said to aid or prevent voice lowering. Probably many of the herbs used to balance hormones, listed under "Estrogen," above, would also be helpful.

WEIGHT CONTROL

✇ CHICKWEED and CLEAVERS help to burn fat. CHICKWEED can be used raw in salads, as capsules, as a tea, or as tincture. Nature's Way Herbal Slim™ prominently features CHICKWEED. As a tea, take three or more cups of these herbs a day, and though it may take up to two months to notice a change, hang in there, for you will notice a considerable change in time.

✇ Many find that YERBA MATÉ, WHITE OAK BARK, or FENNEL will decrease appetite and aid digestion.

✇ HAWTHORN and CHICKWEED tincture in water twice a day are also helpful.

✇ MA HUANG (CHINESE EPHEDRA) and KOLA NUT are thermogenic (persuading the body not to slow its energy burning rate when you cut calories) and are often combined to aid weight loss. HORSE-TAIL is also somewhat thermogenic.[16] It takes about three months for these herbs to really become effective in this capacity. And, like all diet aids, they work best when combined with a sensible diet. CAUTION: EPHEDRA may keep some people awake.

✇ PARSLEY, CORN SILK, or DANDELION are diuretics.

✇ STEVIA is a safe, herbal sweetener.

---

16 Astrup, Arne, "Treatment of Obesity with Thermogenic Agents," *Nutrition* 5(1), January/February, 1989.

❧ ALFALFA is an excellent nutrient, cleanser, and detoxifier, which optimizes the usefulness of other herbs.

❧ FENNEL seed tea is an excellent appetite suppressant. Pour a pint of boiling water over two teaspoons of the seed, cover and let steep 15 minutes. Drink a half a cup or a full cup half an hour or so before meals. You can make this up in larger quantities and store in the refrigerator for up to three days, heating a cupful when you need it or drinking it cold. This is also a good carminative, as is simply chewing a couple of seeds.

❧ CELERY SEED tea is a diuretic, helpful to many who retain water. Crush one or two teaspoons and pour a cup of boiling water over them. Steep ten to 20 minutes. Take two or three cups a day.

❧ CASCARA SAGRADA or other herbs listed under "Constipation" will help to clean out the colon.

❧ BRAN or PSYLLIUM, husks or seeds, or GLUCOMMANAN or GUAR GUM are bulking agents which, when taken with a full glass of water half an hour to an hour before meals will make you feel full so you'll eat less, provide fiber, act as a laxative, and help to stabilize hormones and blood sugar. CAUTION: Do not take bulking agents within an hour of taking vitamins, herbs, or medication. Bulking agents form an indigestible mass, and if your supplements get caught up in it, they pass right on through without helping you at all.

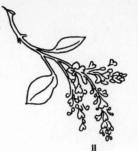

CHAPTER 2

Herbal Notebook

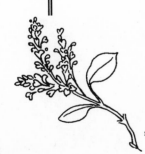

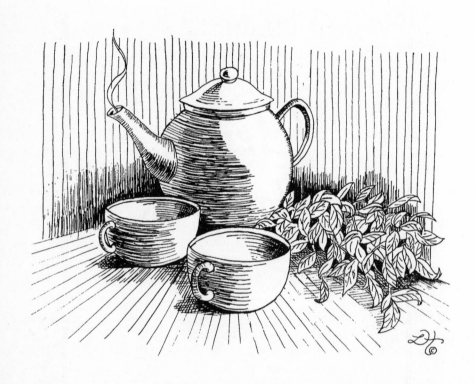

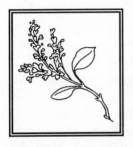 Herbs are so much safer than even the ubiquitous aspirin, that the question of herb safety is almost humorous. While it's true that not all herbs are harmless, neither are all mushrooms. With herbs, as with mushrooms, you need to know what you're doing. WILD HEMLOCK mistaken for WILD CARROT can kill you, and ingesting BEL-LADONNA (*Atropa belladonna*) will just as quickly put out your lights.

But look at the figures. The fact is that thousands of people die or are injured by prescription drugs, household products, and house plants every year. The American Association of Poison Control Centers confirmed in 1991 that there are so few reports of adverse reactions to herbs they don't even have a category in their data-base for herb-related incidents. They do, however, have a large file on poisonings from toxic household and land-scape plants (dieffanbachia, poinsettia, oleander, etc.).[1]

This is not to say that, just because herbs are natural, you need give no thought to their use. Informed common sense is necessary regarding anything you put into your mouth. Too much saturated fat or aspirin can land you in the hospital, as can large doses of LICORICE ROOT if you have high blood pressure. Herbs commonly used today have withstood the test of time. Thousands of years and millions of people have witnessed and documented the safe and effective use of herbs. No other medicine can make that claim.

1 Blumenthal, Mark, *Whole Foods*, 8/91, p. 53.

TEA TERMS

Herbalists prefer to forgo the term "tea" completely for the more specific terms infusion and decoction. These words describe two distinct methods of preparing a tea. Herbalists will say, "Make an infusion of PEPPERMINT" or "Prepare a decoction of WHITE WILLOW BARK." Here's what they mean:

Infusion

This method is preferred for herbs with useful or pleasing volatile oils. As in aroma therapy, part of the desired effect can be due to an herb's agreeable fragrance, such as with PEPPERMINT or EUCALYPTUS. Plants with soft leaves or delicate flowers are also usually prepared as an infusion.

To make an infusion: Place the herbs in a glass or earthenware container that has a close-fitting lid and cover them with the appropriate amount of water which you have just brought to a rolling boil. Allow the herbs to steep in the covered pot for ten to twenty minutes. Then strain out the herbs and either drink or refrigerate the liquid. You can also make an infusion, called "sun tea," by putting herbs and cold water in a clear, covered, glass jar and setting it in the sun for several hours.

Decoction

When the stems, bark, roots, or coarse leaves of an herb contain the healing ingredient needed, the decoction method is preferred.

To make a decoction: Put the herbs in a glass, earthenware, or stainless steel container, cover with water and simmer, uncovered, for about an hour, or until the water is decreased by about half. If the herbs contain valuable volatile oils, the container is covered as it gently simmers. Cinnamon bark would be one example of such an herb.

How Much Herb to Use?

Teas for medicinal use are prepared stronger than for beverage purposes. Most tea bags, for example, contain about only a fraction of an ounce of the herb or herbs, an amount meant for six to eight ounces of water. When infusing or decocting medicinal teas, use one full ounce of a dried herb for each pint (two cups) of water. Since that much dry plant material will absorb some of the water, you'll usually end up with about one and a half cups of liquid. This will normally be enough for three doses, or a day's worth of herbal magic.

If using fresh herbs, double the amount of the herb per pint of water. Dried herbs are "condensed," so to speak, because their water content is zero.

If teas are not your "bag," or if the herb called for is mucilaginous (slimy or slippery when wetted), or you're going to have to be taking a treatment for a long time, you may prefer to use the herb in the form of a tincture, extract, or gelatin capsule.

HOW TO MAKE YOUR OWN
TINCTURES, SALVES, LINIMENTS, POULTICES, OILS,
FOMENTATIONS, AND PILLS

Tinctures

Useful for herbs that don't taste good, for herbs that may need to be preserved almost indefinitely, for herbs to be taken over a long period of time, for herbs containing ingredients not easily extracted by water, or when you want to take a number of herbs and just can't face all those capsules every day. Tinctures might be described as alcohol or vinegar infusions.

To make a tincture: Place about four ounces of the herb, dried or fresh, into a pint of ninety-proof alcohol. Vodka, gin, rum, whiskey, or brandy will suffice. Cover the container, which, by the way, should be glass, and shake it daily for two weeks or so. Then pour off the tincture into another jar or bottle (preferably dark), straining out the herbs through a fine cloth or other filter. A filter used for coffee will work fine. Purists and astrologers (not that they're mutually exclusive!) will tell you that you should begin this process at the time of the New Moon and strain it at the Full Moon. The waxing Moon will help to "draw out" or extract the herb's healing properties.

One generally takes but a small amount—from several drops to a tablespoon or two—of tinctures, but if you wish to avoid even that amount of alcohol, you may substitute pure APPLE CIDER VINEGAR. Another way to eliminate the alcohol is to stir your tincture dosage into a half cup or so of boiling water and let it set for a few minutes. The alcohol should evaporate.

If you can't wait two weeks: Place the herbs in a coffee or other filter, pour a pint of alcohol over the herbs and let it drip, through the filter, into a clean jar or glass coffeemaker container. You can use the tincture after the first dripping, but, of course, the more often you do it, the stronger the tincture.

Fluid Extracts

These are concentrated tinctures, prepared commercially using a multiple extraction procedure. They are usually anywhere from five to ten times stronger than tinctures, and their dosage is correspondingly lower. Follow dosage instructions carefully.

How to Make Salves or Ointments

First, make an herbal oil by gently heating the herb or herbs in oil until the plant loses its color. Then, strain out the herbs and add melted beeswax (about 1½ ounces to a pint of oil) so that the mixture, once it cools, will not be liquid at room temperature. ALMOND OIL, WHEAT GERM OIL, OLIVE OIL, PEANUT OIL, or VITAMIN E OIL are recommended, but use whatever you have (except mineral oil). Liquefied anhydrous LANOLIN oil is good, too, but some people are allergic to it. Add a small amount of VITAMIN E OIL or gum benzoin or tincture of gum benzoin to preserve the salve.

Some people, especially in the "old days," used pork lard, instead of oil and beeswax. You simply macerate the herbs, fresh or dried, and stir them into the melted lard. The mixture is simmered until the herbs become crisp. It is then strained and allowed to cool.

Liniments

Liniments are used most often for sore joints, arthritis, inflammation, strained ligaments, or sore muscles, and usually contain some sort of stimulating herbs combined with antispasmodic herbs. Essential, aromatic oils are usually present, also, to aid in penetration and aroma.

To make a liniment: Add four ounces dried herb, or eight ounces of a fresh herb, to a pint of ALCOHOL, VINEGAR, or OIL. ALMOND, SESAME, PEANUT, or OLIVE OILS are good choices, separately or in any combination. Preserve oil liniments by adding about 400 I.U.s of Vitamin E per eight ounces of oil. The alcohol may be gin or vodka or, strictly for external use only, rubbing alcohol. An alcohol-based liniment will be somewhat cooling when applied. A vinegar-based liniment is astringent, and oil-based liniments are handy when you wish to massage the affected area.

Seal the container and let it sit from 3 to 14 days, shaking it a few times a day. The shorter time is adequate for powdered herbs, while the longer is necessary if using whole herbs or pieces of root or bark. Strain the liquid and add from 10 to 30 drops of an essential oil of your choice, such as WINTERGREEN or EUCALYPTUS.

Poultices

Poultices are used to draw out fever, infection, inflammation, toxins, even foreign matter (such as splinters), to break up congestion, heal bruises, allay spasms, and reduce pain. Poultices are essentially crushed, pulverized, or mashed wet herbs applied directly to the affected area, or folded in a clean cloth and then applied. You may apply them cold or cool to draw off the heat of inflammation or congestion, or warm or hot for spasms or some pains. If the fresh herb is used, it is usually wet enough after crushing, but poultices may be moistened with water, tinctures, infusions, oils, decoctions, or salves.

The appropriate herb is selected according to its healing properties. CABBAGE, for instance, draws toxins from the body. Simply wash a leaf of it, pulverize it, or, at least, crush or break its ridges or veins (perhaps with a rolling pin), and apply it to infected sores, boils, or even to tumors. Hold it in place with a clean cloth or bandage. When the leaf gets warm or hot, replace it with another. COMFREY is known for reducing swellings and healing cuts, open sores, abrasions, or other wounds. Wash the area, apply a warm COMFREY poultice (moistened with COMFREY infusion or other infusions or oils if desired or necessary), and stand by for a miracle. GINGER, CAYENNE, or PRICKLY ASH added to a poultice will promote (healing) circulation to the area.

Essential Oils

You can make your own essential oils, using one of several methods, though they will not be as concentrated as those purchased in a health food store. To use these purchased oils therapeutically, add from ten drops to one ounce of the essential oil to one or two cups of another oil of your choice: SESAME, SUNFLOWER, and WHEAT GERM OIL will be absorbed rather quickly and easily into the skin; while ALMOND, PEANUT, OLIVE, and AVOCADO oils will remain on the skin longer.

To make essential oils: To two ounces of finely crushed herb, add one pint of good oil (OLIVE, ALMOND, etc.) and heat slowly on top of stove or in an oven at 200 degrees or less, until the herbs become crisp. This may take from two to four hours. Strain the oil into a dark jar or bottle.

Another method is to fill a jar loosely with herbs or flower petals of your choice, singly or in combination. (LAVENDER, CHAMOMILE, or ELDERBERRY flowers, plus ROSE PETALS is a nice combination.) Pour oil slowly over the herbs, getting rid of air bubbles, then put the lid on. In warm weather, you can set this jar on a window sill in the sun for 4 or 5 days (maybe less if it's really hot). In cool weather, you may have to let it sit for 14 or 15 days. Shake the jar each day. Then strain the oil into a sterilized bottle or jar.

How to Make Garlic Oil and Garlic Syrup

Peel and mince, or put through a garlic press, four to eight ounces of fresh garlic. Put it all into a sterilized, wide-mouthed jar and cover with OLIVE OIL. Put lid on tightly and let it set from three to seven days. Shake it every day. Then strain off the oil into a dark jar or bottle and store in a cool place. This oil is wonderful for salads, not to mention a host of ailments, including ear infections (two or three drops of the warmed oil in the affected ear two times a day), and even ear mites in pets.

For GARLIC syrup, peel and mince one pound (yes, pound) of garlic and place into a jar. Cover with three parts of APPLE CIDER VINEGAR to one part water. Shake and let set for three or four hours. Strain off the liquid and add an equal amount of honey. Cover, keep in a cool place, and take a tablespoon three to seven or eight times a day for conditions of the lungs (including asthma, congestion, and bronchitis), coughs, poor circulation, cholesterol, poor digestion, and heart weakness.

Fomentations

This is practical way to apply infusions or decoctions to the body. You simply soak a clean, natural fiber cloth or towel in an infusion as hot as the patient can stand it, wring it out gently, and apply to the appropriate area. This cloth is then covered, these days, with plastic wrap. The plastic is topped with a dry towel or cloth and, sometimes, a heating pad. This treatment is useful to stimulate circulation of the blood or lymph, to relieve colic or gas pains, to warm joints, and to reduce internal inflammations. It is said that alternating hot and cold fomentations will bring activity to any area—the kidneys or bowels, for instance—and improve circulation.

Pills

There are advantages to making your own pills. For one thing, there are no fillers which manufacturers use either to bind tablets together or to insure that herbs are free-flowing enough to be used in capsule-filling machinery.

Another advantage, especially if you are a vegetarian, is that you can ensure that you ingest no animal products. "Gelatin" capsules are now available in vegetarian form, but they're more expensive than the ordinary, animal-product, gelatin capsules. Which brings us to a third advantage: it's much cheaper to make your own.

To make pills: Grind your herbs as finely as you can, using either a blender, food processor, coffee grinder, or mortar and pestle. Add a little SLIPPERY ELM powder or some other mucilaginous herb (maybe about a tenth of the whole concoction) and just enough water to make a paste-like texture to hold everything together. Form into pills about the size of a pea. These may be used immediately or dried by spreading them out at room temperature, or you can preheat an oven to 250 degrees, turn the oven off, and place the pills on a plate in the oven for 15 to 30 minutes. Check them often. Bottle, label, and keep them in a dry, cool place.

GELATIN CAPSULES—HOW DO YOU FILL THEM AND WHAT DO THOSE NUMBERS MEAN?

The numbers "00" (double ought) and "0" (single ought) refer to the size of the capsule. Though there are other sizes, these are the most popular. Of these two, the larger one, "00," is usually preferred, unless you find the size difficult to swallow.

How to Swallow Capsules

Do not tilt or throw the head back, as in swallowing tablets. Capsules are light and will float to the back of your throat for easy swallowing if you incline your head slightly forward as you drink. You should drink at least one-half to one cup of liquid when you take capsules in order to assure they're easily dissolved.

How to Fill a Capsule

First, the herb or herbs should be ground to a very fine powder. You may do this yourself, using a blender and then a mortar and pestle, or you may purchase the herbs already powdered. Next, place the powder in a bowl or cup, then take the capsule apart and repeatedly push the open end into the powder. Almost fill both pieces of the capsule, or, if you wish, completely fill the large end only. The powder will pack into the capsule. Rejoin the two pieces and that's all there is to it.

One teaspoon of herb powder will generally fill two "00" capsules, depending on the fineness of the powder and how tightly it's packed into the capsule. One ounce of powder will fill about 40 to 50 "00" capsules or between 50 and 70 "0" capsules.

Dose: The usual recommendation for capsules is two capsules, three times a day. This will vary according to the herb involved, of course, and with your own needs.

Some people may object to gelatin capsules because they are made from an animal product. Capsules made from vegetarian sources are now available, or you may elect to make your own herbal pills.

HERBAL PROPERTIES—HOW TO DESCRIBE
WHAT HERBS DO

ADAPTOGENS help the body to adapt to and cope with all kinds of stressors; improve stamina and resistance and, some say, longevity.

ALTERATIVES purify the blood and thereby encourage and abet the cleansing activities of the detoxifying organs of the body: the liver, kidneys, spleen, and intestines. Alteratives are best used over a long period of time to promote gradual detoxification.

ANODYNES help reduce pain and discomfort.

ANTIBIOTICS destroy and inhibit the growth of bacteria; strengthen the body's immune system.

ANTIPYRETICS cool; reduce or prevent fever; or the term may allude to neutralizing harmful acids in the blood, thus "cooling" it.

ANTISEPTICS prevent the growth of bacteria.

ANTISPASMODICS halt or reduce spasms of the muscles, cramps, and convulsions.

ANTITUMOR (DISCUTIENTS) dissolve and eliminate tumors and growths.

APERIENTS soften the stools; mild laxative effect.

APHRODISIACS are used to correct conditions of sexual imbalance, which, thereby improving over-all health, may induce sexual excitation.

AROMATICS are herbs with a pleasant fragrance and sometimes a pungent taste.

ASTRINGENTS reduce bleeding and inflammation, diminish mucus discharge, increase tissue tone.

CARDIACS strengthen the heart.

CARMINATIVES expel gas from gastrointestinal tract, stimulate peristalsis, thereby firming the internal musculature.

CATHARTICS are laxatives, rapidly empty bowels.

CHOLAGOGUES promote bile production.

DEMULCENTS soothe irritation.

DIAPHORETICS increase perspiration; influence whole circulatory system.

DIURETICS increase urine output, thus they help get rid of water retention; usually combined with Demulcents to allay any urinary tract irritation.

EMMENAGOGUES help to promote menstrual flow, but should be used with care and to promote normal flow, only. Excess dosage could lead to too heavy a flow and possibly extreme discomfort. Will also allay cramps. Unless the herb also falls into the Tonic category, an emmenagogue should not be used during pregnancy.

EMETICS induce vomiting, usually in large doses, usually in tincture or tea form.

EMOLLIENTS are softening and soothing to the skin.

EXPECTORANTS help to expel mucus from throat and lungs; usually combined with Demulcents.

FEBRIFUGES reduce fevers.

GALACTAGOGUES increase secretion of mother's milk.

HEPATICS tone, strengthen, and stimulate the secretions of the liver.

HEMOSTATICS stop internal bleeding.

HORMONAL AGENTS contain ingredients (hormone precursors) the body can use to produce hormones or which can serve as a substitute for the hormones. Many tonic herbs contain hormonal agents, but some non-tonic herbs do, too.

IMMUNE ENHANCERS strengthen the immune system, purify the blood, and can be antiseptic, antibiotic, and antifungal.

LITHOTRIPTICS get rid of kidney and gall stones.

LYMPHATICS cleanse and stimulate lymphatic system.

NERVINES produce sedative-like action, calming and relaxing.

OXYTOCICS promote labor and easy childbirth.

PARASITICIDES kill and eliminate parasites.

SEDATIVES; see Nervines.

SIALAGOGUES promote saliva production.

STIMULANTS arouse or quicken the normal functional activity of the body; boost energy.

STOMACHICS encourage and strengthen functions of the stomach, promoting digestion and appetite.

TONICS strengthen and buoy the whole system, increasing energy and helping it to better cope with stressors of all kinds.

VULNERARIES aid in healing wounds and burns, actually promoting cellular growth and inhibiting infection.

HOW TO CHOOSE AN HERBAL PROPERTY
FOR YOUR NEEDS

Herbal properties can be divided into three main categories, depending on the fundamental effects they produce in the body. Some herbs fall into more than one category; it depends upon how they're used, i.e., strength, frequency, length of treatment.

For Detoxifying

Alteratives
Aperients
Cathartics
Cholagogues
Discutients (antitumor)
Diuretics

Emetics
Expectorants
Laxatives
Lithotriptics
Lymphatics
Parasiticides

For Symptom-relief

Anodynes
Antibiotics
Antipyretics
Antiseptics
Antispasmodics
Carminatives
Demulcents
Diaphoretics
Emetics

Emmenagogues
Emollients
Febrifuges
Hemostatics
Mucilages
Oxytocics
Sedatives
Sialagogues
Stimulants

For Toning and Building

Aphrodisiacs
Astringents
Cardiacs
Diaphoretics
Emmenagogues
Galactagogues
Hepatics

Nervines
Nutritives
Oxytocics
Stomachics
Tonics
Vulneraries

SOME HERBS AND THEIR PROPERTIES

With this information and the information in "Herbal Properties," you can mix and match herbs to suit your needs. For example, for PMS, you might choose to combine herbs from the following categories: diuretics, hormonal agents, nervines, anodynes, sedatives, and tonics.

BARBERRY: Antiseptic, hepatic, stomachic, alterative, aromatic, tonic, lithotriptic, immune enhancer.

BLACK COHOSH: Antispasmodic, expectorant, emmenagogue, diaphoretic, cardiac, alterative, tonic.

BLACK WALNUT: Antiseptic, astringent, antifungal, alterative, antitumor, lymphatic, parasiticide.

BLESSED THISTLE: Emmenagogue, galactagogue, stomachic, tonic, alterative.

BLUE COHOSH: Antispasmodic, emmenagogue, oxytocic, diuretic.

BUCHU: Antiseptic, diuretic, diaphoretic, lithotriptic.

BURDOCK ROOT: Alterative, diaphoretic, diuretic, demulcent, antitumor, nutritive tonic, antipyretic, antibiotic, aphrodisiac, hormonal agent, stomachic, carminative, astringent, urinary tonic, tonic.

BURDOCK SEEDS: Alterative, diuretic, tonic, demulcent, vulnerary, relaxant.

BURDOCK LEAVES: Tonic, cholagogue, diuretic, vulnerary, antitumor.

CALENDULA: Astringent, vulnerary, antispasmodic, diaphoretic.

CATNIP: Carminative, diaphoretic, sedative, febrifuge, nervine.

CAYENNE: Carminative, stimulant, antispasmodic, astringent.

CHICKWEED: nutritive, restorative, hormonal agent, antipyretic, alterative, carminative, demulcent, emollient, vulnerary.

CELERY: Carminative, diuretic, nervine, stimulant, tonic .

CHAMOMILE: Emmenagogue, nervine, sedative, carminative, diaphoretic, tonic, anodyne.

CHAPARRAL: Alterative, antibiotic, antiseptic, lithotriptic, antitumor, parasiticide, lymphatic, emetic.

CHASTEBERRY: Hormonal agent, tonic, emmenagogue.

CLEAVERS: Alterative, astringent, diuretic, antipyretic, laxative, immune enhancer.

COMFREY: Demulcent, expectorate, mucilage, vulnerary, alterative, astringent, nutritive.

CORNSILK: Diuretic, lithotriptic, demulcent.

CRAMPBARK: Antispasmodic, astringent, nervine.

DAMIANA: Emmenagogue, tonic, aphrodisiac, cholagogue, diuretic.

DANDELION FLOWERS: Anodyne, emollient, vulnerary, hepatic, calmative, cardiac.

DANDELION LEAVES: Nutritive, tonic, galactagogue, stomachic, cholagogue, aperient, diuretic, vulnerary, anodyne, febrifuge.

DANDELION ROOT: Hepatic, cholagogue, lithotriptic, tonic, nutritive, galactagogue, digestive, stomachic, aperient, laxative, diuretic, astringent, antifungal, antibacterial, sedative.

DEVIL'S CLAW: Alterative, antitumor, lithotriptic, stimulant.

DONG QUAI (*Angelica sinensis*): Emmenagogue, hormonal agent, uterine tonic, antispasmodic, alterative.

ECHINACEA: Alterative, antiseptic, lymphatic, parasiticide, sialogogue, immune enhancer.

FALSE UNICORN ROOT: Emmenagogue, tonic, diuretic, emetic, parasiticide, stimulant.

FENUGREEK: Demulcent, emollient, expectorant, aphrodisiac, astringent, galactagogue, hormonal agent, tonic.

GARLIC: Alterative, antibiotic, antispasmodic, diaphoretic, expectorant, stimulant, lymphatic, immune enhancer, parasiticide.

GINSENG (PANEX): Alterative, stimulant, stomachic, tonic, cardiac, liver tonic, hormonal agent, immune enhancer.

GINSENG (SIBERIAN): Adaptogenic, antispasmodic, cardiac, tonic, hormonal agent, immune enhancer.

GINKGO: stimulant, improves circulation, especially to the brain. It is a rich source of antioxidants.

GOLDENSEAL: Alterative, antibiotic, antiseptic, emmenagogue, stomachic, tonic, laxative, immune enhancer.

GOTU KOLA: Nervine, tonic, alterative, antipyretic, diuretic.

HAWTHORN BERRIES: Tonic, antispasmodic, cardiac, astringent, diuretic, sedative.

HOPS: Nervine, stomachic, anodyne, antibiotic, carminative, cholagogue, tonic.

HORSETAIL: Astringent, diuretic, lithotriptic, emmenagogue, galactagogue, nutritive, vulnerary.

IRISH MOSS: Demulcent, emollient, nutritive.

JUNIPER BERRIES: Antispasmodic, diuretic, anodyne, aromatic, astringent, carminative, lithotriptic, stimulant.

KELP: Demulcent, nutritive, alterative, diuretic, antitumor, antitoxic, antiradiation, antistress, antibiotic, cardiac, aphrodisiac, aperient, anodyne, nervine, immune enhancer, calmative.

LICORICE ROOT: Demulcent, expectorant, laxative, alterative, hormonal agent, immune enhancer.

LOBELIA: Antispasmodic, emetic, nervine, expectorant.

MARSHMALLOW (*Althea officinalis*): Demulcent, diuretic, emollient, lithotriptic, alterative, nutritive, vulnerary.

MOTHERWORT: Emmenagogue, nervine, tonic, cardiac, antispasmodic, diaphoretic, laxative.

MYRRH: Antiseptic, emmenagogue, carminative, expectorant, stimulant, immune enhancer.

NETTLE LEAF: Nutritive, tonic, galactogogue, anti-anemic, diuretic, laxative, lithotriptic, alterative, antiseptic, antidiabetic, antirheumatic, astringent, antiasthmatic, expectorant, hemostatic (the fresh juice).

NETTLE SEED: Antiseptic, rejuvenative, vermifuge, laxative, antitoxic (poison antidote).

NETTLE ROOT: Tonic, astringent, diuretic.

OATS and OATSTRAW: Nervine, tonic, antispasmodic, demulcent, antidepressant, antidiabetic, febrifuge, diuretic, diaphoretic, carminative, stimulant, aperient.

OREGON GRAPE ROOT: Alterative, cholagogue, laxative, tonic, lithotriptic, lymphatic.

PARSLEY: Diuretic, carminative, expectorant, nervine, tonic, lithotriptic.

PASSION FLOWER: Antispasmodic, sedative, diaphoretic, nervine, anodyne, aperient.

PAU D'ARCO: Alterative, antifungal, antidiabetic, bitter tonic, digestive, antibiotic, antitumor.

PENNYROYAL: Diaphoretic, emmenagogue, antispasmodic, carminative, stimulant.

PEPPERMINT: Aromatic, carminative, diaphoretic, stimulant, antispasmodic.

PLANTAIN: Diuretic, emollient, alterative, antiseptic, astringent, expectorant, vulnerary, aperient.

POKE: Alterative, lymphatic, antibiotic, anti-inflammatory; emetic and cathartic in large doses but not recommended; best combined in small doses with other herbs.

RASPBERRY LEAF: Antispasmodic, astringent, alterative, stimulant, tonic, hemostatic, anodyne.

RED CLOVER: Alterative, nutritive, sedative, stimulant, antitumor, antispasmodic, expectorant.

ROSEMARY: Aromatic, carminative, diaphoretic, stimulant, astringent, antipyretic, anti-inflammatory, stomachic, nervine, anodyne, antiseptic.

RUE: Antispasmodic, emmenagogue, stimulant.

SAGE: Antispasmodic, astringent, aromatic, vulnerary.

SARSAPARILLA: alterative, carminative, tonic, hormonal agent, diaphoretic.

SAW PALMETTO: Diuretic, tonic, antiseptic, sedative, hormonal agent, aphrodisiac.

SKULLCAP: Antispasmodic, nervine, antipyretic.

SHEPHERD'S PURSE: Astringent, diuretic and urinary antiseptic, hemostatiatic, stimulant.

SLIPPERY ELM BARK: Demulcent, emollient, nutritive, astringent.

SQUAW VINE: Emmenagogue, astringent, diuretic.

SUMA: Energy tonic, adaptogen, demulcent, nutrient, hormonal agent, anodyne.

UVA URSI: Astringent, diuretic, alterative, antiseptic, tonic

VALERIAN ROOT: Antispasmodic, nervine, carminative, stimulant, sedative, anodyne.

VIOLET: Demulcent, expectorant, alterative, antipyretic, antiseptic, vulnerary, antispasmodic, antitumor.

WHITE OAK BARK: Astringent, antiseptic, diuretic.

WILD YAM: Cholagogue, antispasmodic, diaphoretic, expectorant, hormonal agent.

WILLOW BARK: Anodyne, antispasmodic, tonic, astringent, diaphoretic, diuretic, febrifuge.

WITCH HAZEL: Astringent, hemostatic, anti-inflammatory, tonic, sedative.

WOOD BETONY: Nervine, alterative, aromatic, liver tonic, sedative, parasiticide,

YARROW: Astringent, diaphoretic, hemostatic, stimulant, antispasmodic, stomachic, antipyretic, carminative, urinary tonic, febrifuge.

YELLOW DOCK: Alterative, astringent, cholagogue, laxative, nutritive, lymphatic.

KINETIC TESTING FOR PRODUCT
SELECTION AND DOSAGE

Sometimes called muscle testing, this is an incredible technique you probably won't believe until you try it. It's a way of determining what your body needs at the moment and how much it wants.

There are two techniques, each very simple, but each requiring the help of a loyal assistant. After you've located your helper, here's what you do.

First, extend your left arm and hold it horizontally, perpendicular to your body. Ask your assistant to press down on your extended arm, saying, "Resist me, (your name)." This determines your base-line strength. Your helper should not apply all of his or her strength in trying to lower your arm. This is just to get a feel for your "normal" strength.

Next, hold a bottle of herbal capsules or vitamins or a food in your right hand against your chest, and perform the above extended-arm procedure again. Your assistant should say something like, "Testing (product) to see if it's what (your name) needs at this time." Or say nothing at all. Do as you like. If, while holding the substance, your resistance is weaker, even by a little, this is not the product for you at this time. If you're the same or stronger, your body can benefit from this product at the moment. If you're *really* stronger, your body is saying, like Audrey II to Seymour in *The Little Shop of Horrors*, "Feed me! Feed me!"

Don't believe it? Want to test the test, first? OK. Skeptics are welcomed here. Try the experiment with something you know is not good for you, say, a box of sugar or candy, a pack of cigarettes, or whatever. Unless you're wasted away to practically nothing or your adrenals are exhausted (in either case, your body will take anything it can get), you'll markedly weaken when tested with the "no-no" product.

A similar method involves holding the thumb and forefinger of the left hand together at the tips and having a friend try to part them while you hold the product to be tested in your right hand. Remember, this is not a test of who's stronger, you or your friend, but a test of your own relative strength.

To determine dosage, hold a fairly large amount of the item in your right hand to start with. Begin with a handful of capsules and have your friend say something like, "We're now testing to see how much (your name) needs to take per day." You'll probably test weak with the handful. Have your friend remove one capsule at a time, testing and repeating the sentence after each removal until you reach your ideal dose.

ALL ABOUT DONG QUAI— A WOMAN'S WONDER HERB

DONG QUAI (*Angelica sinesis, A. acutiloba*) has come through at least 2,000 years of extensive clinical experience. Chinese medical texts dating back that far repeatedly mention DONG QUAI (also known as "tang-kuei") and its many benefits for practically every complaint known to woman. It has survived scrutiny in the "scientific era," as well. It has been found that DONG QUAI:

Nourishes female glands
Regulates menses
Rebuilds blood
Helps the mother after birth of a baby
Allays hot flashes and cramps
Allays PMS

In addition, it is often combined with other herbs and taken by both men and women for:

Skin diseases, especially eczema
Hypertension
Kidney disorders (including nephritis)
Candida (fungus) infections
Tumors
Diabetes

Cancer
Angina pectoris
A tonic

It has been demonstrated to be an effective antibacterial, antifungal, immunostimulant (causing interferon production), and antitumor agent. It's also a good source of Vitamin B12.

Depending on preparation methods, DONG QUAI can be used either to stimulate or to relax the uterus. A decoction prepared over a long period of time (to get rid of its volatile oils) stimulates the uterine muscle to contract. A decoction of DONG QUAI prepared in a shorter time, using low heat, prompts the uterus to relax. DONG QUAI can also regulate uterine function, and is therefore useful to treat profuse menstruation.

In laboratory experiments, animals given DONG QUAI exhibit higher DNA content in their uteri, plus a higher rate of glucose metabolism. This would help explain DONG QUAI's ability to heal uterine tissue.

DONG QUAI is usually taken in capsules or brewed as an infusion or decoction. For many women, two capsules a day is plenty, though the tonic dose recommended by herbalists is from four to eight capsules a day. Listen to your own body's wisdom. Kinetic testing is also useful. For acute ailments, 12 to 20 capsules per day are recommended. For PMS and menopausal symptoms, a typical course of treatment is to take DONG QUAI for seven to ten days, usually during the latter part of the cycle (after ovulation or when ovulation would have occurred), during the months you feel you need help. Or, see above for decoction preparation methods for specific results.

GARLIC—WHAT SCIENTISTS SAY

Here's what scientists have lately confirmed about the pharmacological properties of GARLIC:[2]

1. Lowers serum total and low density lipoprotein cholesterol in humans.

2. Raises high density lipoprotein cholesterol (HDLs), in humans.

3. Reduces the tendency of blood to clot, and the aggregation (i.e., clumping) of blood platelets.

4. Modulates the conversion of arachidonic acid (A.A.) to eicosanids, thereby inhibiting inflammation.

---

2 From *Herbal Healthline*, Volume 2, Number 2, 1991, edited by Dr. Michael A. Weiner, Ph.D., p. 8.

5. Inhibits cancer cell formation and proliferation by inhibiting nitrosamine formation, modulating the metabolism of polyarene carcinogens, and by acting on cell enzymes which control cell division.

6. Protects the liver from damage induced by synthetic drugs and chemical pollutants.

7. Kills intestinal parasites and worms, as well as gram-negative bacteria.

8. Protects against the effects of radiation.

9. Offers anti-oxidant protection to cell membranes.

10. Researchers make no mention of the literary tradition that garlic can keep vampires away.

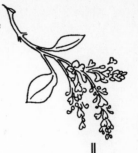

CHAPTER 3

Vitamins & Minerals for Menopause

*We should study nature more, and act
according to nature, whose rules are few,
plain and most reasonable.*
— William Penn

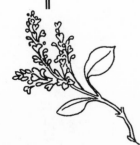

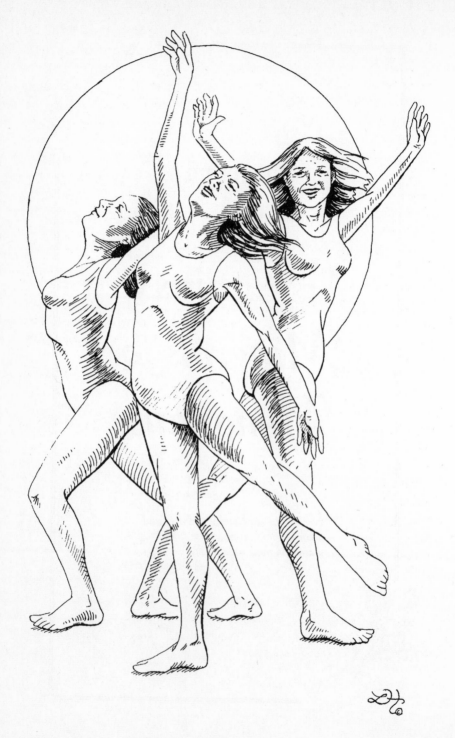

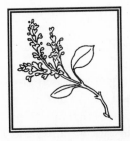

Vitamins are not drugs or medicine, nor are they just "pills" or supplements to be taken in lieu of eating properly. Vitamins are substances found in our foods that are vital to our health and growth. Vitamins occur in foods in relatively minute quantities (compared to fats, proteins, and carbohydrates). Without them, though, our bodies cannot function properly, and we become susceptible to all manner of mental and physical ills.

In fact, life cannot be sustained without vitamins, which, but for a few exceptions, we must obtain from foods or from supplements, since our bodies do not produce them.

Vitamins are like fuel additives necessary to operate our bodies. Enzymatic processes cannot function without vitamins and minerals, and enzymatic processes regulate and balance the over-all functioning of our magnificent machine. A deficiency of even one vitamin can disrupt the beautiful order and precision that should prevail.

Unfortunately, in these days of refined, processed, and long shelf-life "fresh" foods, not even a "balanced" diet can provide all the nutrition necessary. Even if it did, our relatively sedentary lifestyles dictate that we eat a correspondingly low-calorie cuisine, and this, in itself, limits vitamin intake. It is no secret, however, that most Americans, generally opting more for convenience and personal taste preferences than for nutrition, do not eat a balanced diet. The situation has little improved since 1972 when Dr. Jean Meyer, then of Harvard's Department of Nutrition, and Chairman of the 1969 White House Conference on Food, Nutrition and Health, informed us that: "Malnutrition, whether caused by poverty or improper diet, contributes to the alarming health situation in the United States . . ."[1]

---

1 *Science*, April 21, 1972.

Even those who somehow manage to get the USDA's Minimum Daily Requirement (MDR) or Recommended Daily Allowance (RDA) are not achieving their optimum health potential. Wrote Senator William Proxmire of Wisconsin, in a 1974 issue of *Let's Live*: "At best the RDAs are only a 'recommended' allowance at antediluvian levels designed to prevent some terrible disease. At worst they are based on conflicts of interest and self-serving views of certain portions of the food industry. Almost never are they provided at levels to provide for optimum health and nutrition."[2] It is really no wonder we could all benefit from vitamin and mineral supplementation.

"But," you say, "most of the foods I eat are fortified and enriched with vitamins and minerals. It says so right on the box."

Fortified, indeed. If I were to take $20.00 from you and then give you back $3.00, would you feel enriched? That's exactly how your foods are "enriched." Twenty-two naturally occurring nutrients are removed or destroyed in the processing of breads and cereal grains, for instance, and then six or so are put back in. Often, as in the case of IRON, these "enriching" nutrients are in a form that is not readily assimilated by the human body. In the case of milk, the synthetic VITAMIN D added to it depletes the body of MAGNESIUM,[3] which, in addition to VITAMIN D and other nutrients, is essential for the optimum utilization of CALCIUM. MAGNESIUM and CALCIUM are important for heart, muscle, and nerve functioning, as well as for bones and teeth. (It may seem strange, but minerals are also nutrients for our bodies and play an important role in enzymatic processes.)

At menopause, whether naturally or artificially induced, with our bodies going through transformations comparable in scope and stressfulness to the changes that occurred at puberty, our body's demand for the proper fuel and fuel "additives" is dramatically increased. Whether acknowledged by the medical mainstream or not, today *there is a large and growing body of research supporting the benefits of vitamin and mineral supplementation* (sometimes in so-called megadoses—which may actually be "normal" doses—the RDAs being so low!), for menopause and beyond. There are also first-hand experiences of our sisters who've been through it. Let us listen to them—and to ouselves.

---

2 Passwater, Richard A., *Supernutrition*, Pocket Books, New York, 1975.

3 Mindell, Earl, *Vitamin Bible*, Warner Books, New York, 1985.

ARTHRITIS/JOINT PROBLEMS

Almost 50 percent of all women report some form of joint problems upon approaching and entering menopause. Often, the proper supplements can prevent or alleviate the arthritis-like symptoms.

❧ A deficiency of SELENIUM, a trace mineral and ANTIOXIDANT, has been implemented in the development of the pain and swelling of arthritis. Other ANTIOXIDANTS are usually taken with SELENIUM, especially VITAMINS C and E, because they facilitate its absorption. SELENIUM is called a trace mineral because our bodies require only relatively minute amounts. SELENIUM is usually taken in amounts ranging from 50 to 200 micrograms a day. (A microgram is 1/1000 of a milligram, or, to put it another way, one millionth of a gram.)

❧ DL-PHENYLALANINE (DLPA), pronounced fennel-AL-ah-neen, is a unique mixture of a synthetic (D) and naturally occurring (L) form of the amino acid, PHENYLALANINE. It is both a remarkable painkiller and an antidepressant. It is not habit-forming like many modern painkillers, is nontoxic, and it is excellent for chronic pain. It does not need to be increased over time, because the body does not build up a tolerance or resistance to it as it does to morphine or other drugs used for chronic pain; it helps many people when other pain-relievers won't, and it does not interfere with medications or other therapies. It works by stimulating the production of the body's own painkilling resources, morphine-like hormones known as endorphins.

DLPA's effects usually take three or four days to kick in, though in some people relief is immediate. In some cases, relief may take up to three weeks to be felt. If after three weeks, you notice no improvement, double the dose for another three weeks. If there is still no effect, quit using it. It doesn't work for about 15 percent of the population. Dosage, to begin with, is usually 750 mgs. about 15 minutes before each meal. It should not be taken with milk or other protein drink, nor with a meal. After improvement is noticed, you can gradually reduce the dosage until you find the amount your body requires for mainte-nance. Some people need to take it only a few days every few weeks for continued relief. Some take one or two capsules a day for maintenance. You should find your own level.

CAUTION: It can raise blood pressure, so if yours is high already, monitor yourself carefully. Some people with hypertension can still take DLPA if they take it after meals. Pregnant persons or people with

PKU (phenylketonuria—an allergy to PHENYLALANINE) should not take either DLPA or L-PHENYLALANINE.

✿ 3000 TO 6000 mgs. of VITAMIN C per day. Spread the dosage. VITA-MIN C has many useful properties, one of which is as an anti-inflam-matory agent and another is its role in the production of collagen, the stuff that holds you together and is the padding between some joints and the vertebrae. Another of VITAMIN C's helpful traits is that it helps you cope with stress, and if you're in pain, you're under even more stress than the average person. Aspirin, by the way, depletes the body of VITAMIN C. VITAMIN C is water soluble and must be replaced daily; we do not manufacture it for ourselves, nor can we store it. It is "used up" as it does its various jobs throughout the body.

✿ Take a 100 mg. B-COMPLEX three times a day. Stress eats up those B VITAMINS, too!

✿ Extra VITAMIN B12, up to 2000 mcg (MICROgrams) a day, may also help. You can get it in a form to be taken under the tongue (sublingual) from health food stores these days. B12 is difficult to absorb orally, especially for some people and especially as we get older. That's why it's usually given as an injection. The sublingual form, with sorbitol (a natural sweetener) is apparently absorbed quite well.

✿ Extra NIACIN (in addition to what's in the B COMPLEX tablets) is often of assistance, as well. Spread the dosage and be prepared for some skin flushing, at least in the beginning. Don't go overboard, though. Too much NIACIN is hard on your liver.

✿ A good multi-vitamin and mineral tablet or capsule in addition to everything else.

✿ Cod liver oil (VITAMIN A, OMEGA-3 FATTY ACIDS) is also a good addition to your anti-arthritis regimen. It seems to especially help rheumatoid arthritis. In its emulsified, flavored liquid form, it's really not that bad tasting. Take a tablespoon on an empty stomach an hour before breakfast, an hour before lunch, or just before bedtime or all three. Skip two days a week.

✿ Salmon oil capsules (OMEGA-3 FATTY ACIDS) also apparently help a number of people, especially with rheumatoid arthritis. Some have found relief taking anywhere from three to six capsules three times a day.

CONCEPTION AND CONTRACEPTION

Improving your health by supplying your body with all the nutrients it needs and craves will improve both your sexuality and your ability to conceive. If you want to avoid conception, menopause is no excuse to let your guard down. Ovulation can occur without warning even after months of inactivity. As mentioned in Chapter One, after one year with no periods, especially after age 52, conception is unlikely, but not impossible. Conventional oral contraceptives are not recommended for optimum health, however.

The Pill robs your body of VITAMINS B6, B12, FOLIC ACID, and VITAMIN C. Depression is just one of the common side-effects of the Pill. Why? VITAMIN B6 is necessary for TRYPTOPHAN metabolism, and, if you're on the Pill, your need for B6 is 50 to 100 times that of someone who doesn't take oral contraceptives. It's doubtful you obtain that much B6 daily, unless you take a very potent supplement. And what does TRYPTO-PHAN do? It is an amino acid used by the brain to produce the neurotransmitter, SEROTONIN. Serotonin has a calming effect, and a lack of it can result in various sleep disorders, depression, and irritability. VITAMIN B6 is also important in the synthesis of DNA and RNA, NUCLEIC acids which help keep us young, energetic, and sexy.

CONSTIPATION

⅋ A B-COMPLEX deficiency can be implicated in poor bowel function.

⅋ VITAMIN C, complex carbohydrates, pectin, and ACIDOPHILUS foster the growth and maintenance of friendly bacteria in our intestines. This promotes colon health, digestion, and proper elimination.

⅋ 8–10 glasses of water a day, plus fiber, plus exercise, are also necessary to prevent constipation.

DEPRESSION, NERVES, IRRITABILITY

⅋ VITAMIN C is helpful in some cases of depression, especially if one of the symptoms is a dry mouth.[4] It helps you deal with stress, in any case, and keeps the immune system boosted.

---

4 Enwonwu, C. O., "Hypfunction of Salivary Glands in Ascorbic Acid Deficiency," *Medical Science Research*, 18:353-354, 1990; Fackelmann, K. A., "Vitamin C May Reduce Hypertension Risk," *Science News*, May 12, 1990; Murray, Frank, "Vitamin C. Deficiency Causes Health Problems," *Better Nutrition*, November, 1990.

❧ DLPA (DL-PHENYLALANINE), an amino acid, is a safe and effective antidepressant. L-PHENYLALANINE also does the job. Please see cautions and details under ""Arthritis," above.

❧ Another amino acid, TYROSINE, is an antidepressant. TRYPTOPHAN is, too, if you can get it. (See "Insomnia," below, for a discussion of tryptophan.)

❧ A goodly supply of the B COMPLEX daily will prevent or alleviate depression. B6 is especially important, here, as it assists the brain in converting TRYPTOPHAN into SEROTONIN. (See "Conception.") A lack of VITAMIN B1 can also lead to depression. Sugar and alcohol severely deplete the body of these vitamins. If you heavily indulge in either as a rule—or even "binge" once in a while—try VITAMIN B COMPLEX for a change. Your outlook will greatly improve. Incidentally, it is not a good idea to take large amounts of just one or two of the B VITAMINS for an extended length of time. Take the whole complex at the same time. For depression take a 100 mg. B COMPLEX VITAMIN three times a day. B VITAMINS are water soluble and nontoxic.

❧ VITAMINS B5 (PANTOTHENIC ACID) and B12 can help you deal with stress and will probably give you some energy, too. Be sure to take them with the rest of the B COMPLEX. For best absorption of B12, take it in the sublingual form.

❧ "The Pill" can cause depression, as can beta blockers, synthetic estrogens, drugs for high blood pressure, arthritis, and a host of other drugs. If you're taking any medications, ask your doctor or pharmacist about their side effects or read up on them yourself. There are a number of books on the subject; check your local library.

❧ MAGNESIUM, 400–500 mg. per day, balanced with twice as much CALCIUM, can alleviate depression, especially if you happen to be deficient in this important mineral. Both CALCIUM and MAGNESIUM are natural tranquilizers and painkillers. MAGNESIUM also "feeds" your nerves. If you are taking estrogen or the birth control pill, you require larger than average doses of MAGNESIUM.

❧ LECITHIN granules aid in efficient brain and nerve performance; one or two tablespoons once or twice a day are helpful in some cases of depression. CAUTION: LECITHIN should not be taken during the depressive stage of manic depression. It may deepen the depression in this case.

ENDOMETRIOSIS

Menopause itself usually cures this problem, but, as menopause is a process usually occurring over several years, you may find one or more of the following helpful in the meantime.

🎐 EVENING PRIMROSE OIL, BORAGE OIL, BLACK CURRANT OIL, SALMON OIL, or other sources of OMEGA-3 and/or OMEGA-6 fatty acids, which decrease inflammation, can be helpful for this condition.

🎐 VITAMIN E, BETA CAROTENE, and VITAMIN C should help to decrease the inflammatory response. They'll also aid in the healing process, as will ZINC.

ENERGY

🎐 RNA and DNA supplements are said to be rejuvenating and energizing after a couple of months, taken as follows: one 100 mg. tablet a day for one month, then two per day for another month, then three per day from then on for six days a week. These nucleic acids can also be obtained in wheat germ, bran, spinach, asparagus, mushrooms, fish, oatmeal, brewer's yeast, chicken liver, and onions.

🎐 The B COMPLEX VITAMINS are necessary for energy production.

🎐 POTASSIUM-MAGNESIUM ASPARTATE can apparently increase energy and endurance. It also enhances fat-burning.

🎐 VITAMINS B5 (PANTOTHENIC ACID) and B12 will help you fight fatigue. Be sure you take the complete B COMPLEX along with them. For best absorption of B12, use the sublingual (under the tongue) form, 1000–2000 mcgs.

ESTROGEN, HORMONE BALANCE

🎐 In studies of post-menopausal women, supplementation of 3 mg. of the trace mineral BORON increased the level of a beneficial form of estrogen (estradiol 17B) in the blood by 50 percent. Though BORON is found in apples, grapes, pears, and nuts, the surest way to know you're getting enough is to take one 3 mg. supplement daily.

🎐 VITAMIN E, in doses of 400 IU to 1600 IU daily alleviate menopausal symptoms for many women, especially hot flashes. CAUTION: If you have high blood pressure, begin VITAMIN E supplementation at 100 or 200 IUs and work up slowly to a higher dosage.

❧ The B VITAMINS, particularly B6, are beneficial in a hormone-balancing program. A good place to start is 50 to 100 mg. of the B-COMPLEX, with 100 to 200 mg. additional B6. Play with the dose until you find the one that is right for you.

❧ VITAMIN F, particularly from EVENING PRIMROSE OIL (EPO), BLACK CURRENT OIL, or other sources of GAMMA LINOLENIC ACID is a powerful hormone balancer. Two capsules of EPO three times a day might prove a useful dose.

❧ Some foods and herbs supply estrogen-like substances and estrogen precursors used by your body to produce estrogen. See the appropriate chapters.

FIBROIDS

Menopause usually shrinks, if not eliminates, fibroids. While it's in the process of working this wonder, though, the following will also help the situation.

❧ Again, a good vitamin/mineral supplementation program is beneficial. This should include 50 to 100 mgs. of the B COMPLEX, with an additional 100 to 200 mg. of VITAMIN B6.

❧ VITAMIN E, a valuable ANTIOXIDANT, has been found extremely useful in eliminating lumps of the breast. Over the course of a month or so, gradually work up to a maximum dose of 1000 IUs of VITAMIN E a day, then reduce the dosage to 600 to 800 IUs a day. If the fat-soluble E is not to your liking, a dry form is available. WARNING: VITAMIN E is essentially nontoxic, but should be used with caution if you have an overactive thyroid, diabetes, high blood pressure, or rheumatic heart disease. If so, begin with a very low dose and gradually work up to 100 IUs a day per month, continuing, also gradually, up to a maximum of 400 to 800 IUs per day. If you decide to decrease your dose, do that slowly, too.

❧ COENZYME Q10, another ANTIOXIDANT, is useful to take in conjunction with VITAMIN E.

❧ EVENING PRIMROSE OIL or other sources of GAMMA LINOLENIC ACID, also known as VITAMIN F, is also beneficial. Two capsules three times a day is a possible dose.

❧ Eliminating caffeine and, for some people, dairy products, helps, too.

HAIR

Gray Hair

✿ PABA (Para-aminobenzoic Acid), a member of the B-COMPLEX group, familiar as a sun-screening agent, has been reported by some people, including famed nutritionist, Adelle Davis, to restore gray hair to its natural color. Along with good overall nutrition and the other B VITAMINS, take 300 to 500 mg. of PANTOTHENIC ACID, 5 (five) mg. of FOLIC ACID, some INOSITOL, and 300 mg. of PABA per day.[5] Others suggest simply 1000 mg. of PABA a day six days a week. Downside: when you quit the regimen, the gray comes back; plus, high dosages of PABA may result in nausea and vomiting in some people. CAUTION: Don't take PABA if taking methotrexate (Mexate), a cancer drug. PABA and FOLIC ACID may inhibit effectiveness of sulfa drugs.

✿ BIOTIN, a member of the B COMPLEX, deters graying.

✿ Gray hair has also been produced (experimentally, in animals) by a COPPER deficiency, as well as by a deficiency of the above-mentioned VITAMINS. CAUTION: Supplementing with COPPER is not usually recommended (depletes ZINC stores and may lead to other health problems). Just eat plenty of whole grains, green leafy vegetables, and liver.

Falling hair

✿ B COMPLEX, twice a day.

✿ A chelated multi-mineral complex once a day, making sure you get a total of 1000 mg. of CALCIUM and 500 mg. of MAGNESIUM per day, either included in the mineral complex or taken in addition to the complex to total that amount.

✿ VITAMIN C, 500 mg. six times a day, or 1000 mg. three times a day.

✿ CHOLINE and INOSITOL, 1000 mg. each per day.

✿ Without sufficient VITAMIN A, your hair can become dull and lifeless and will eventually fall out. A tablespoon of emulsified, flavored cod liver oil a day is good for skin, hair, and many of our other parts. Take it on an empty stomach, at bedtime or an hour before breakfast.

---

5 Davis, Adelle, *Let's Get Well*, Harcourt, Brace, Jovanovich, New York, 1965, p.138.

(Emulsified and flavored, it isn't bad. Really.) Allow about six weeks or so for the first glimmering of results.

Healthy Hair

&a VITAMIN F, or unsaturated fatty acids, promote healthy, glossy hair. You should have twice as much unsaturated fatty acids in your diet as you do saturated fats. Never cut out all fats and oils from your diet.

&a The regimen listed under "Falling Hair" is a good prescription for healthy hair in general. As a maintenance program, though, you could reduce the B COMPLEX dosage by half, taking it only once, instead of twice, a day.

&a Also add, or make sure your multiple vitamin contains, CYSTEINE, one of the amino acids. Take a total of 1000 mg (1 gram) daily, between meals with water or juice and your VITAMIN C.

&a Also add a multivitamin, once a day.

HEADACHES, MIGRAINE, OR OTHER

Fluctuating hormone levels produce headaches in some 70 percent of women approaching or going through the menopause. Avoid over-the-counter painkillers as much as you can and try some of the following. Supplements listed under "Estrogen," should help, too.

&a NIACIN, a B VITAMIN, VITAMIN B3, taken with the complete B COMPLEX, plus CALCIUM and MAGNESIUM has been found effective for many types of headaches, including chronic ones. Fifty to 100 mg. of NIACIN is taken three times a day. This amount of NIACIN will cause flushing for a few minutes (a bit like a hot flash). Some report that this flushing ceases after you've taken NIACIN for a while. CAUTION: If you have severe diabetes, glaucoma, peptic ulcers, or impaired liver function, you should use NIACIN cautiously. Don't take timed-release NIACIN, however. Some recent research indicates it could cause liver problems.

Take a timed-release B COMPLEX of 100 mg twice a day, plus 1000–1500 mg of CALCIUM and 500–700 mg. of MAGNESIUM. Take the CALCIUM and MAGNESIUM in two or three doses; they're very tranquilizing and may make you too sleepy if the total amount is taken all at once. CALCIUM and MAGNESIUM are also painkillers.

❧ DLPA (DL-PHENYLALANINE), an amino acid, is effective against headaches, including migraines, especially of the chronic variety. For most people, it won't work as well as aspirin, getting rid of a headache on an occasional, acute-treatment basis. Please see cautions and further explanation of DLPA under "Arthritis," above.

HEART PALPITATIONS

It can be very strange and scary to feel your heart pulsating rapidly. Many women experience this at sometime during the menopausal years. Fortunately, several natural aids are available, the key being, once again, adequate nourishment for this all-important muscle and your entire body. In this day and age of high stress levels and during the added stress of menopause, "adequate" nutrition, more often than not, means taking in much more than the standard RDAs and MDRs. The following regimen should help.

❧ Again, take a good (strong) multi-vitamin and mineral, making sure to get about 1000 mg CALCIUM and 400–500 mg MAGNESIUM. (If you live in an area where the water is hard, you may not need quite that large a dose of calcium and magnesium. Studies have shown that people in hard water areas have healthier hearts than those who drink soft water.) A deficiency of MAGNESIUM has been implicated in arrhythmia (irregular heart beat). Both minerals are necessary for proper muscle functioning.

❧ One hundred mg timed-release B COMPLEX, twice a day.

❧ Nine to 18 LECITHIN capsules a day, in divided doses, or one to three tablespoons of the granules.

❧ At least 3,000 mg. of VITAMIN C, in divided doses.

❧ VITAMIN E, approximately 400 IUs a day, aids both the heart and circulation. One study at Harvard University of 87,245 female nurses who took more than 100 IUs of VITAMIN E a day for more than two years demonstrated a 46 percent lower risk of heart attacks![6]

❧ An inadequate intake of SELENIUM has been implicated in an increased risk of heart problems.[7] It is an important ANTIOXIDANT which prevents the formation of harmful FREE RADICALS. One hundred to 200 mcgs. have been recommended.

---

6 *Whole Foods,* 1/93, p. 27.

7 Kok, Frans J., Ph.D., et al. "Decreased Selenium Levels in Acute Myocardial Infarction," *Journal of the American Medical Association,* February 24, 1989.

HOT FLASHES AND NIGHT SWEATS

This old standby for stand-up comedians is no joke. They do eventually go away after a few years, but who wants to wait when you can do something to prevent or greatly reduce them? Here are some choices:

§ VITAMIN E in the amount of 400 IUs, one to four times a day, eliminates hot flashes for a great many women. CAUTION: Start slowly, using the lower amount for a few days and gradually working up to a dose high enough to stop your hot flashes, if you have high blood pressure. VITAMIN E can temporarily raise blood pressure when you first start taking it. One woman I know (who did not have high blood pressure) took one VITAMIN E capsule of 1000 mg. once a day for a few days. It completely eliminated the hot flashes she was experiencing about every fifteen minutes, which, she said, were driving her (and her family) crazy. After that she just took one every other day and remained symptom free. *This is not a recommended procedure,* but she was obviously desperate. Again, one should begin with small doses and gradually work up to higher ones. Please see WARNING, under "Fibroids," above.

§ A high potency (100 mg. or more) VITAMIN B COMPLEX taken twice a day, along with 1000 mg. of VITAMIN C with 500 mg. of the BIOFLAVONOIDS (including about 50 mg. of RUTIN and HESPERIDIN) three times a day, plus a strong multi-vitamin and mineral tablet helps relieve or prevent many of the symptoms of menopause, including hot flashes. The minerals should be chelated (KEE-lated); this improves their absorption.

§ HESPERIDIN, in dosages of 1000 mg a day, has been shown to relieve hot flashes.

INSOMNIA

About 50 percent of women find that at sometime during the menopause they have trouble sleeping. It is ironic, when you consider that there are finally no crying babies or late-coming-home teenagers in the house anymore, and you really *could* sleep now, if only you could.

§ CALCIUM and MAGNESIUM capsules or tablets (you can get them combined in the proper ratio of twice as much CALCIUM as MAGNESIUM) three times a day, for a total of about 1000 mg. of CALCIUM, plus three tablets taken half an hour or so before bedtime.

CALCIUM and MAGNESIUM are natural tranquilizers without the adverse side-effects of strong sedatives and hypnotics, such as pheno-barbital, Nembutal, Butisol or other drugs often prescribed by doctors. CALCIUM and MAGNESIUM have the added benefits of aiding heart, muscle, nerve, and bone health.

✖ If the amino acid TRYPTOPHAN is ever allowed back on the market by the FDA, it is an excellent—and safe—insomnia-chaser. It has been used harmlessly by millions for years. It was taken off the market sev-eral years ago, amidst much media ballyhoo, when several people con-tracted Eosinahilia Myalgia Syndrome, a rare blood disorder, after taking TRYPTOPHAN. Unfortunately, there was no matching bally-hoo in the media when the source of the problem was identified: one contaminated batch of TRYPTOPHAN from one Japanese company. Even though the problem was with only one batch and the situation was corrected, the FDA still (as of 1994) won't allow it to be sold. If they ever do, the dose is about 500 to 700 mg. taken an hour to an hour and a half before bedtime with juice or water (not milk). It works best when taken with VITAMIN B6, NIACINAMIDE (a non-flushing form of NIACIN), and MAGNESIUM. Meanwhile, TRYPTOPHAN is found in turkey, chicken, bananas, milk, and some other protein foods. How about a turkey sandwich and a glass of milk before going to bed?

✖ One hundred mg. of VITAMIN B6 and of NIACINAMIDE will help you reach your goal of a good night's sleep. Together, they stimulate the production of the brain chemical, SEROTONIN. The B6 may stim-ulate dreams, too. A good time to start a dream diary?

INVOLUNTARY, FREQUENT, OR BURNING URINATION

✖ Enhancing your estrogen level can often prevent or cure this problem because a drop in the amount of estrogen in the body can thin the ure-thra, allowing a reduction in the urine-retaining pressure of that tube. Vaginal walls get thinner, reducing their ability to support the urethra, also. Therefore, the methods for increasing and maintaining estrogen in your system will be useful here, unless the problem is due to some other cause. See measures listed under "Estrogen."

MEMORY

ॐ L-PHENYLALANINE, an essential amino acid, can improve both your mental alertness and memory. Take it between meals with water or juice. A protein, such as milk or a soy-based drink, interferes with its effectiveness. It *can* raise blood pressure and those with PKU should not take it. Please see DLPA under "Arthritis," for cautions and more details.

ॐ LECITHIN will also help to improve the memory and mental alertness. Studies done on college students demonstrated that those who took LECITHIN while studying for a test and just before the test did better than those who didn't take LECITHIN. A tablespoon or more of the granules daily is a good dose. It takes care of cholesterol and aids heart and circulation, too.

ॐ CHOLINE (kole-leen), part of the B COMPLEX, found in small amounts in LECITHIN, also aids memory, and assists nerve impulses. PHOSPHATIDYL CHOLINE (fos-feh-tidal kole-leen) is the most bioavailable form.

ॐ TYROSINE (TIE-roe-zeen), an amino acid, is found in dairy foods, egg yolks, and animal flesh. If you've been cutting back on these foods and have noticed yourself becoming especially forgetful or "scatter-brained," this may be just what you need. Take one 500 mg. supplement in the mornings and you'll enjoy enhanced memory, thinking, and concentration all day.

MENSTRUATION

ॐ VITAMIN B6, a good diuretic, also appears to aid the body in handling raging, or even non-raging, hormones, helping to alleviate PMS symptoms. It also appears to decrease estradiol (estrogen) and increase progesterone levels. A dose of from 50 to 300 mg. a day, starting a few days to two weeks before one's period and continuing throughout the period, has helped many women, though some find it necessary to take as much as 150 mg. three times a day. Start with the lower dose and increase to the higher over the course of a week or more. This should be accompanied by a 100 mg. B-COMPLEX morning and night, or even three times a day, as well as your usual (strong) multi-vitamin and mineral tablets and your VITAMIN C (1000 mg. three or four times a day), of course. A high dosage of a single B VITAMIN should never be taken by itself over any extended length of time. It should be taken in conjunction with the whole B COMPLEX, or else certain B-VITAMIN deficiencies could result, rather spoiling the whole effect you were aiming for in the first place.

❧ CALCIUM and MAGNESIUM are often helpful, but, oddly enough, during the PMS phase, it is sometimes more helpful to reverse their usual two-to-one ratio. Experiment to see if that procedure helps you. Try 500 mg. MAGNESIUM, and 250 mg. CALCIUM a day, or even two or three times that amount if necessary. Take these two freely for pain, too, if necessary, instead of over-the-counter painkillers. If you're craving chocolate, sugar, or salt, you probably need more CALCIUM, MAGNESIUM, or ZINC, or all three.

❧ To further aid CALCIUM absorption, make sure you get at least 400 IUs of VITAMIN D and 3 mg. of BORON daily.

❧ VITAMIN C with BIOFLAVONOIDS in 1000 to 3000 mg. (divided) doses will help you cope. To slow heavy flows, take it to the point of bowel tolerance (diarrhea begins), then cut back, but don't stop taking it.

❧ VITAMIN E can be useful here, too—100 to 400 IUs will usually do the trick.

❧ Extra ZINC, 30–50 mg. per day, at this time appears to help some women.

❧ One of the B VITAMINS, extra PANTOTHENIC ACID may help, in amounts up to 1000 mg. a day.

❧ EVENING PRIMROSE OIL, though not strictly a vitamin, does supply the polyunsaturated fatty acids, GAMMA LINOLENIC ACID (GLA) and LINOLEIC ACID (LA), which are important in the production of beneficial prostaglandins, which in turn help with symptoms of PMS and menopause. (Unsaturated fatty acids are sometimes called VITAMIN F.) Today's diets and lifestyles have a tendency to interfere with our ability to convert essential fatty acids into GLA.

❧ NIACINAMIDE has helped to control PMS-related sensitivity in some women.

❧ VITAMIN C and NIACIN help cramping and "nerves."

🏵 DLPA (dl-PHENYLALANINE), started a week to ten days before the expected period or whenever you begin to feel those warning signs indicating your period (or the time when you'd normally have a period if you've already stopped them or become irregular) is great for mood and pain. Please see DLPA under "Arthritis," above for cautions and more detail on its use.

🏵 Try to do something almost every day to work up a sweat, and have at least one good laugh a day.

OSTEOPOROSIS

All of the following deplete your bones of CALCIUM: fluoridated water, alcohol, sedentary lifestyle, smoking, soft drinks, excess caffeine, high-protein meat diets, cortisone, anticoagulants, anti-seizure drugs, liver or kidney malfunctions, poor digestion, low-estrogen. Plus, with age, our need for CALCIUM to build our bones increases. Time to start shoring up the defenses, wouldn't you say?

🏵 VITAMIN C, 3000 mg. or more per day, 400–800 IUs of VITAMIN E, 100–200 mcg. of SELENIUM, 50 mg. of ZINC, 400–800 IUs of VITAMIN D, and all the vitamins and minerals, actually, are important for bone health, many playing a part in effective CALCIUM assimilation.

🏵 A digestive enzyme helps assimilation of the pertinent nutrients, especially hard-to-digest minerals. Try BETAINE HYDROCHLORIDE or PAPAYA or others.

🏵 BORON, a trace mineral, is important for the proper utilization of CALCIUM and thus for bone health. Given 3 mg. of BORON a day, post-menopausal women not only demonstrated enhanced CALCIUM uptake, but also 50 percent more estrogen in their systems. Increased estrogen availability, of course, also aids CALCIUM use and in so doing can prevent or reverse osteoporosis. Researchers think BORON is used in the actual production of estrogen, VITAMIN D, and other hormones and in preventing their rapid deterioration in the body.

🏵 MAGNESIUM aids in the absorption of CALCIUM as well, so, it, too, is important to bone health. Take half as much MAGNESIUM as you do CALCIUM daily.

🏵 GERMANIUM will help to alleviate bone pain.

❧ MANGANESE, another trace mineral, is also necessary for healthy bones. A high intake of CALCIUM and PHOSPHORUS may increase the need for this mineral. Only 4 or 5 mg. are needed per day, however; and it can generally be easily obtained from food, depending on the MANGANESE content of the soil they were grown in.

❧ SILICON is another mineral that will help you maintain strong bones. Kelp, algaes, and hard water are good sources.

❧ To speed healing of broken bones: increase CALCIUM intake up to 1500 mg and VITAMIN D up to 500 IUs a day.

SEX

A well-nourished body is the best aphrodisiac there is. It's reported that 20 percent of menopausal women experience a decrease in sexual desire. One wonders what better nutrition might do for them. Or the other 80 percent! Try the following and find out for yourself.

❧ L-PHENYLALANINE has been known to increase a person's interest in sex. It should be taken between meals with water or juice. Please see DLPA under "Arthritis," for cautions and details.

❧ VITAMIN E, 400 IUs, anywhere from one to three times a day. See cautions under "Heart," above.

❧ ZINC, 30 to 50 mgs, one to three times a day.

❧ A good multiple vitamin/mineral supplement once or twice a day.

❧ VITAMIN B COMPLEX, 50 to 100 mg., once or twice a day.

❧ VITAMIN C, with BIOFLAVONOIDS, 1000 mg., three or four times a day.

SKIN

You've heard the expression, "garbage in, garbage out" applied to all sorts of situations. Well, guess what? It also applies to your skin. What goes into your mouth and stomach is more important than what you put on your skin. It is the largest organ you have and needs nourishing just like the rest of your body. One of the most helpful things you can do for your skin is to drink six to eight glasses of water a day.

Dry Skin

⁊ VITAMIN C deficiency can lead to several problems, including dry skin.

⁊ VITAMIN E oil helps immensely. Take it internally and apply it to the skin. You can buy VITAMIN E oil in bottles or you can puncture a capsule with a pin and squeeze it out. This could get quite tedious if you need to cover a large area, obviously. VITAMIN E oil is very soothing and healing for burns and, applied faithfully to a wound or incision for some time, will prevent scars or even eliminate old ones.

⁊ VITAMIN A and VITAMIN D, both applied and ingested, will also aid dry skin. You wouldn't want to apply cod liver oil (!), but taking a tablespoon of the emulsified, flavored version of this old standby once a day will benefit dry skin and hair. Cod liver oil, of course, is a good source of VITAMIN A. Take it on an empty stomach an hour before breakfast or just before bedtime. Allow six to eight weeks for results to be noticed. For VITAMIN A capsules, you may want to try 25,000 IUs (international units) a day for a few weeks, then cut back to 10,000 IUs a day for maintenance. Listen to yourself; you'll know. The more you listen and heed yourself, the more you *will* know, the more reliable your "gut feelings" will be.

⁊ Get adequate VITAMIN F, unsaturated fats, either in the form of supplements (EVENING PRIMROSE OIL, BLACK CURRANT OIL, LINSEED OIL—not the hardware store kind!) or make sure you're getting twice as much unsaturated fats as saturated fats in your diet. Unsaturated fats come from plant sources, including nuts and seeds. (Coconut and palm oils, however, are saturated.) Never eliminate all oils and fats from your diet. You'll dry up and look like a prune, and many bodily functions will not work right. VITAMIN E, taken with VITAMIN F in any form, aids its absorption.

Healthy, Glowing Skin

⁊ B COMPLEX tablet, taken after a meal, once a day. 100 mg., timed release.

⁊ VITAMIN C, at least 3000 mg. a day. You can take a 1000 mg. tablet after each meal or take six 500 mg. tables, spread out through the day. This is easy to do if you carry some chewable C around in your pocket. Many nutritionists maintain that you get more benefit from C if it's taken in small, multiple doses. (The FDA notwithstanding, I consider 500 mg of C a small dose for an adult.) If the acidity of C bothers you, get the buffered or acid-free kind, or take it with some CALCIUM.

❧ VITAMIN A, 25,000 IU of it or of BETA CAROTENE. Skip two days a week on this one, although BETA CAROTENE is okay daily. BETA CAROTENE is a precursor of VITAMIN A; it is converted to VITA-MIN A in your body only up to the amount your body needs.

❧ VITAMIN E, one to three 400 IUs daily. An easy way to remember is to take one after each meal. You're not skipping any meals, are you?

❧ One thousand mg. of CHOLINE and INOSITOL a day, or two table-spoons of LECITHIN granules.

❧ BIOTIN, one of the B VITAMINS helps keep skin healthy and has been used in the treatment of skin problems, including eczema.

❧ CHLOROPHYLL is an excellent system purifier and antibiotic. It's available in liquid or capsule or tablet form. A good dose is two to three teaspoons a day in water (take your other supplements with it) or three tablets after each meal.

❧ 1000 mg. of CYSTEINE a day, taken between meals with water or juice.

❧ A chelated multiple mineral tablet, one or two per meal.

❧ Several ACIDOPHILUS capsules with or after each meal is very useful in these days of antibiotic-laced meat and chlorinated water. ACI-DOPHILUS keeps the useful, friendly bacteria in our intestines. This improves digestion, which aids everything, including the skin.

Age Spots

❧ FOLIC ACID, one of the B VITAMINS, taken in doses of from 1 to 5 mg. for a short time may eliminate skin discolorations. If you normal-ly take high doses of VITAMIN C, estrogen, aspirin, or if you drink much alcohol, your need for FOLIC ACID is increased. Adequate FOLIC ACID is necessary for a strong immune system, too.

Wrinkles

❧ Supplementation with RNA and DNA, called NUCLEIC ACIDS, have decreased wrinkles and sagging after a couple of months. DNA-RNA supplements are available from health food stores. A recommended dose is one 100 mg. tablet a day for a month, then two a day for a month, then three a day from then on. Skip one day a week. These NUCLEIC ACIDS can also be obtained in wheat germ, bran, spinach, asparagus, mushrooms, brewer's yeast, fish, oatmeal, chicken liver, and onions.

❧ The ANTIOXIDANTS, VITAMINS A, C, D, E, SELENIUM, and GERMANIUM are all said to help prevent wrinkles because of their free radical scavenging activity. For the same reason, they're effective anti-aging factors in general. They also protect us against pollution and radiation.

❧ PABA, 30 to 100 mg. taken three times a day is said to prevent or delay wrinkle formation.

VAGINAL DRYNESS

❧ BORON, since it raises the level of estrogen in the blood, may alleviate vaginal dryness. It is thought that BORON is involved in the production and preservation of estrogen. A supplement of 3 mg. per day is all that is required.

❧ VITAMIN E suppositories inserted into the vagina take care of this problem, even better than estrogen creams. Insert one suppository vaginally nightly for six weeks, then use one weekly or as needed. The J. R. Carlson Laboratories produce such a product, known as "Key-E Suppositories." Health food stores should be able to get them for you, or, consulting the "How to Make" section in Chapter 2, you could make your own using VITAMIN E oil and slippery elm powder or beeswax.

VARICOSE VEINS

Brought about when valves which normally keep blood from "falling" back and pooling in the veins of the legs collapse, varicose veins are not only unsightly, but also painful. Chronic constipation and lack of exercise are contributing factors. Lack of proper nutrients to keep the veins strong and flexible can be another.

❧ 3000 to 5000 mgs. of VITAMIN C with BIOFLAVONOIDS (especially rutin) a day. Spread the dose throughout the day in 500 or 1000 mg. increments. This will strengthen the blood vessels.

❧ VITAMIN E, starting at 200 to 400 IUs and, in 100 to 200 IU increments per week, gradually working up to 1000 to 1200 IUs daily. CAUTION: Do not begin with this higher amount.

❧ Also take a good, potent dose (50+ mgs.) of the B's two or three times a day.

❧ 10,000 to 25,000 of VITAMIN A and/or BETA CAROTENE.

❧ A good multi-vitamin/mineral (combined or separate), making sure it contains MANGANESE, SELENIUM, and SILICON.

❧ VITAMIN D, 1000 IUs.

❧ VITAMIN F, the essential fatty acids, from salmon oil, EVENING PRIMROSE OIL, LINSEED OIL CAPSULES, or BLACK CURRANT OIL.

❧ 50–80 mg. of ZINC.

❧ CALCIUM and MAGNESIUM, 1000–1500 mg and 500–750 mg..

❧ POTASSIUM is also important, about 100 mg. daily.

❧ Get plenty of FIBER in your diet. Exercise!

WEIGHT CONTROL

It's interesting to note that thin women have a more difficult menopause than heavier women. Again, Mother Nature knows best. Did you know that fat cells produce estrogen? Relax and be yourself. Eat right and your body will find its proper weight, no matter what society dictates. But if you feel your weight is a problem, read on.

There can be as many causes for overweight (or under, for that matter) as there are people. Oddly enough, though, one of the main causes of overweight may be malnutrition, whether from poor diet and supplementation, poor absorption, insufficient liver function, or whatever. Your body must have and literally craves the nutrients it needs to operate at its best.

Fat cannot be metabolized or used efficiently without the right nutrients to do the job. In other words, fat cannot be burned if the furnace (the body) is not stoked with the proper fuel it needs to function. It takes energy to burn fat and the output of energy relies on the availability of just about every nutrient that we know of. Skip some, leave some out, skimp on others, the mix just won't work. Like making a cake, if you don't put in the flour, or stir in only half as much as is needed—well, it just won't be cake as we know it.

Likewise, you must mix in every ingredient called for in the original recipe to get us human angel cakes as light as we could, should, or want to be. Did you know, for instance, that inadequate VITAMIN E can reduce fat metabolism by half? That LECITHIN helps to burn fat, but only if sufficient CHOLINE and INOSITOL (two B VITAMINS) are present? If there is insufficient PANTOTHENIC ACID (another B VITAMIN) the utilization of fat is also greatly reduced? The list goes on and on.

So, as your mama always said, "Eat your vegetables! Take your vitamins!"

✌ A good multiple vitamin/mineral supplement is necessary. These are available in tablet, capsule, powder, and liquid forms, so if one kind gives you problems, try another. Always go for quality from a health food store you know and trust to be sure what's on the label is actually in the bottle.

✌ Add a B COMPLEX VITAMIN, 50 to 100 mgs., taken twice a day.

✌ Extra B5 (PANTOTHENIC ACID) will aid the adrenals and fat metabolism. Five hundred mg. per meal will do.

✌ LECITHIN granules, a tablespoon or two a day, or some with each meal, will also help move fat out.

✌ L-PHENYLALANINE, one of the essential amino acids, can be an appetite suppressant. Take one or two tablets an hour before each meal with juice or water. A protein drink, such as milk, interferes with its effectiveness. Please see DLPA under "Arthritis," for cautions and details.

✌ VITAMIN F (Unsaturated fatty acids, i.e., LINOLEIC, LINOLENIC, ARACHIDONIC) aids in the burning of saturated fats, when taken in a two-to-one ratio. That is, twice as much unsaturated fat in relation to saturated fats should be consumed in order to keep burning those saturated fats away. If you eat a lot of carbohydrates, your need for essential unsaturated fatty acids is increased (still in the proper ratio). If you get enough LINOLEIC ACID, the body can synthesize the remaining two. VITAMIN E, taken with VITAMIN F in any form, aids its absorption.

VITAMIN F is readily available in foods such as seeds and nuts (18 pecan halves or 4 tablespoons of sunflower seeds can furnish an adequate daily supply).

It is also found in EVENING PRIMROSE OIL (EPO), BLACK CURRANT OIL, LINSEED OIL, and others. These are available in capsule form. EVENING PRIMROSE OIL and BLACK CURRANT OIL supplements are rather expensive compared to, say, VITAMIN C, so if you come across some that are very cheap—no matter what it says on the label—call or write the company and ask for independent assay information confirming that their product does, indeed, contain 100 percent of the particular oil only. Some labels will say, "Contains 100 percent EVENING PRIMROSE Oil," and they are not lying. The EPO in it is 100 percent EPO, but the product may contain only a small amount of it; the remaining contents may be, say, safflower or soy oil. (The same goes for GARLIC OIL capsules, too, by the way.)

✌ CHOLINE aids in fat metabolism. Six LECITHIN capsules contain about 244 mg. of CHOLINE. Two or three times that amount of CHOLINE is often recommended.

✌ DNA–RNA tablets, 100 mg. each, three tablets a day.

✌ VITAMIN E, 400 IU, twice a day. As mentioned elsewhere, if you have high blood pressure, start slowly and gradually increase to your desired dose. VITAMIN E helps speed the rate of fat metabolism.

✌ CHROMIUM PICOLINATE, a trace mineral, 200 mcg (micrograms) a day. Normalizes blood sugar, curbs cravings for sweets, with moderate exercise burns fat, aids thyroid.

✌ VITAMIN C, with BIOFLAVONOIDS, 1000 mg. three times a day, or, better yet, 500 mg. six times a day.

✌ A chelated multiple mineral, twice a day. CALCIUM should total about 1000 mg. for the day and MAGNESIUM, 500 mg.

✌ POTASSIUM-MAGNESIUM ASPARTATE apparently enhances the body's ability to burn fat.

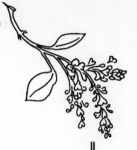

CHAPTER 4

Vitamin & Mineral Notebook

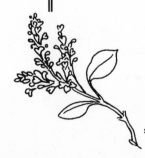

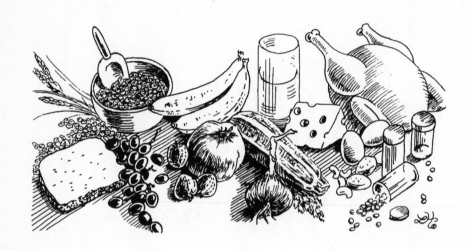

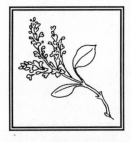 Most vitamins and supplements should be taken with or soon after a meal. Amino acid supplements, however, should be taken between meals with water or juice (not milk) for the best absorption. There are bodily priorities as to what is allowed to cross the "brain barrier" and when. Following these rules takes advantage of these priorities.

❧ Suggested daily amounts should be divided among your meals. (A body can handle only so much at once!)

❧ INORGANIC IRON (ferrous sulfate) should not be taken within eight to twelve hours of taking VITAMIN E.

❧ Synthetic vitamins versus natural source vitamins: though the chemical structure may be identical for each, in some cases, there is significant evidence that the body better utilizes natural vitamins and obtains some additional "unknown factors" that exist in natural products. There is also a synergistic factor among substances that naturally occur together—the VITAMIN C COMPLEX, containing BIOFLAVONOIDS, versus synthetic ASCORBIC ACID, for instance. Yet, when high dosages of vitamins are required to treat an acute disease or condition, the synthetic versions are sometimes necessary. It's difficult to get high dosage amounts of VITAMIN C made from rose hips, for example. ASCORBIC ACID is synthetic VITAMIN C; most B VITAMINS in amounts over about 10 mgs. are synthetic; dl-alpha tocopherol is synthetic VITAMIN E. For maintenance or prophylactic doses, however, the more natural your supplements, the better. (See quote at the beginning of Chapter 3.)

❧ Suggested daily amounts from this book or any other source are just that: *suggested* amounts. The actual amount *you* need will depend on many factors: your age, nutritional status, health status, genetics, amount of pollution you're exposed to, your absorption ability, emotional and physical stresses, the softness or hardness of the water you drink and whether it's chlorinated and/or fluorinated, and the type of foods you eat are some of the factors influencing your ability to utilize vitamin and mineral supplements. Accordingly, some people may require much higher doses than others. This is where paying attention to what your body is telling you, to your intuition, and to how you feel, as well as perhaps doing some kinetic testing, now and again, can be helpful. You are unique. No one, but no one—except you—can tell you what is best for you.

ᴂ Given today's lifestyles, environment, and generally nutritionally deficient foods, one should take supplements daily, probably forever. However, large doses for therapeutic purposes, i.e., to handle a specific disease or condition, should be taken for the duration of that illness only. This is especially true of large doses of single, synthetic B VITAMINS. Long-term use of a single B VITAMIN or two can result in imbalances or even deficiencies of other B VITAMINS.

HOW MANY CARROTS EQUAL A DOSE?

ᴂ To obtain the proven preventative benefits of BETA CAROTENE, you would need to eat 3 to 4 large carrots or 10 cups of broccoli per day.

ᴂ To get VITAMIN C's immune enhancing advantage: 2½ oranges or peppers, or 7 tomatoes each day.

ᴂ For a daily 100 IUs of antioxidant VITAMIN E: 1 pound of almonds, 9+ cups of kale, or 4 cups of olive oil.

ᴂ Bottom line: Food alone won't cut it nutritionally; we just don't eat that much of the right foods. Supplementation alone won't, either— you have to have food. Solution: combine the two for better health.

VITAMIN AND MINERAL TERMS

ᴂ AMINO ACID—the constituent parts of protein. The end result of protein digestion is its breakdown into individual amino acids, which then go scurrying about doing their individual and collective jobs of maintaining our bodies. There are twenty-two amino acids. For adults, eight of these are essential, meaning we must obtain them from sources outside ourselves. For children, there are nine. The remaining, classed as nonessential, can be manufactured within our bodies, given the right nutrients and conditions to do so. Foods which contain all of the essential amino acids are called a complete protein. These include meat and dairy products. Incomplete proteins are missing one or more of the essential amino acids and must be combined with other foods containing the missing nutrients to provide our bodies with a complete protein. Combining beans (legumes) and rice or corn tortillas (whole grains), or peanut butter (legume) and whole-grain bread, are examples of combining foods to obtain a complete protein. (See Chapter 8.) If even one essential amino acid is missing, or is not in correct ratio with the others, protein utilization is impaired and the effectiveness of the remaining essential amino acids is reduced. (This is one reason fad diets restricting certain types of foods and overemphasizing others are not only worthless, but also harmful.)

✤ ANTIOXIDANT—a nutrient that prevents the formation of free radicals by hindering the oxidation (rancidity) of body fats. Free radicals are pesky little devils that are harmful to the body in many ways. ANTIOXIDANTS "scavenge" free radicals, slowing down the aging process.

✤ BIOFLAVONOIDS—Also known as VITAMIN P, which stands for permeability factor. They strengthen capillaries and regulate membrane absorption (permeability). Part of the VITAMIN C COMPLEX, they work synergistically with C, increasing its effectiveness and absorption. They also work with VITAMIN C to promote collagen production and health.

✤ BETA CAROTENE—also known as provitamin A, it is the "precursor" of VITAMIN A found in plant and some animal sources. Your body converts beta carotene into the amount of VITAMIN A it requires at the moment. The orange color in carrots is beta carotene. The term, "beta carotene" is used almost interchangeably with VITAMIN A in much writing. When you read of pumpkin containing VITAMIN A, for instance, the actual substance referred to in this case is beta carotene.

✤ CHELATION—a process which changes minerals into a form more easily digested and absorbed by the human body. These minerals are then called CHELATED. The minerals are often bound to amino acids in this process.

❧ COLLAGEN—the main component of connective tissue, bone and cartilage.

❧ DIURETIC—increases urination, used to eliminate extra fluids from the body.

❧ DNA—deoxyribonucleic acid, a constituent of chromosomes.

❧ ENTERIC COATED—a tablet coated with a substance that resists breaking down in the acid environment of the stomach, waiting to dissolve in the intestines.

❧ ENZYME—a substance in the body that initiates or activates chemical changes; i.e., digestive enzymes chemically alter food so that our bodies can utilize their chemical constituents.

❧ FREE RADICALS—Chemicals produced in the body in response to certain conditions related to oxidation. Free radicals are unstable and steal electrons from other needed chemicals. Thought by many scientists to be instrumental in the aging process and the underlying cause of degenerative diseases, such as cancer, heart disease, and others, they can be controlled by another body of substances called ANTIOXIDANTS. ANTIOXIDANTS prevent oxidation.

❧ IU—international units.

❧ LINOLEIC ACID (VITAMIN F)—one of the polyunsaturated fats, known as an essential fatty acid because it must be obtained from our foods, plus, it is necessary for life itself—for one thing, essential fatty acids are needed for the synthesis of prostaglandins.

❧ LIPID—a fat

❧ LIPOTROPIC—prevents excessive buildup of fats in the liver.

❧ MEGAVITAMIN THERAPY—treating illnesses or health problems with large amounts of vitamins and minerals.

❧ PALMITATE—water-solubolized VITAMIN A.

❧ PKU—phenylketonuria, a condition caused by the lack of the enzyme to digest PHENYLALANINE, an essential amino acid.

❧ PROSTAGLANDINS—one of the substances necessary for hormonal balance. Supplied with the proper nutrients, our bodies produce prostaglandins. VITAMIN F is one of those nutrients.

❧ RDA—Recommended Dietary Allowances, established by the Food and Nutrition Board, National Academy of Sciences, and the National

Research Council as estimates of the amount of nutrients needed by Americans in 1941. They were never intended to be dietary "laws."

❧ RNA—ribonucleic acid, a constituent of chromosomes.

❧ ROSE HIPS—the "seed" of the rose, it is the nodule found beneath the bud. It is a highly concentrated source of VITAMIN C.

❧ TOCOPHEROLS—compounds that make up VITAMIN E (alpha, beta, delta, epsilon, eta, gamma, and zeta), obtained from vegetable oils. Natural source VITAMIN E is designated d-alpha tocopherol, or d-beta tocopherol or whatever. Synthetic VITAMIN E is designated dl-tocopherol, an "L" is inserted after the "D."

❧ TOXIN—an organic poison produced in organisms, whether living or dead.

❧ TRIGLYCERIDES—fatty substances in the blood.

❧ USRDA—United States Recommended Daily Allowance.

FOOD AND HERBAL SOURCES OF VARIOUS VITAMINS AND MINERALS

Vitamins

❧ A: dandelion, cod liver oil, liver, carrots, green and yellow vegetables, eggs, dairy products, yellow fruits.

❧ B COMPLEX: dandelion, whole grains, animal flesh and products, seeds, nuts, some fruits and vegetables. (See individual B VITAMINS.)

❧ B1, THIAMINE: brewer's yeast, brown rice (it's in the husks, discarded from white rice), whole wheat, oats, peanuts, pork, many vegetables, bran, milk.

❧ B2, RIBOFLAVIN: milk, liver, kidney, brewer's yeast, cheese, leafy green vegetables, fish, eggs.

❧ B3, NIACIN: liver, lean meat, whole wheat, brewer's yeast, kidney, wheat germ, fish, eggs, roasted peanuts, poultry's white meat, avocados, dates, figs, prunes.

❧ B5, PANTOTHENIC ACID: whole grains, wheat germ, bran, meat, kidney, liver, nuts, chicken, brewer's yeast.

❧ B6, PYRIDOXINE: brewer's yeast, bran, wheat germ, liver, kidney, heart, cantaloupe, cabbage, blackstrap molasses, milk, eggs, beef.

❧ B12, COBALAMIN: liver, beef, pork, eggs, milk, cheese, kidney, comfrey, soy beans.

❧ BIOTIN: nuts, fruits, beef liver, brewer's yeast, egg yolk, milk, kidney, brown rice.

❧ CHOLINE: egg yolks, heart, brain, liver, lecithin (a little), green leafy vegetables, wheat germ, brewer's yeast.

❧ FOLIC ACID: leafy greens, watercress, parsley, chicory, dandelion, amaranth, lambsquarters, whole grains, dark green leafy vegetables, carrots, torula yeast, liver, egg yolk, cantaloupe, apricots, pumpkins, avocados, beans.

❧ INOSITOL: brewer's yeast, liver, dried lima beans, beef brains, beef heart, cantaloupe, grapefruit, raisins, wheat germ, blackstrap molasses, peanuts, cabbage.

❧ PABA: liver, brewer's yeast, kidney, whole grains, brown rice, wheat bran, wheat germ, molasses.

❧ C: dandelion, citrus fruits, tomatoes, green and leafy vegetables, potatoes, sweet potatoes, berries, cauliflower.

❧ D: dandelion, cod liver oil, other fish liver oils, sardines, herring, salmon, tuna, dairy products.

❧ E: oats, wheat germ, soy beans, vegetable oils (processed without heat), broccoli, Brussels sprouts, leafy greens, whole grains, eggs.

❧ F, UNSATURATED FATTY ACIDS: vegetable oils: wheat germ, linseed, sunflower, safflower, soy bean, peanut; nuts, seeds, avocados.

❧ K, MENADIONE: oats, yogurt, alfalfa, egg yolk, safflower oil, fish liver oils, kelp, leafy green vegetables, soy bean oil.

❧ P, BIOFLAVONOIDS: the white inner skin and interior membranes of citrus fruits; apricots, buckwheat, blackberries, cherries, rose hips.

Minerals

❧ BORON: leafy vegetables, pears, apples, nuts, grapes; best bet: 3 mg. daily supplement.

❧ CALCIUM: dandelion, oats, dairy products, soy beans, sardines, salmon, peanuts, walnuts, sunflower seeds, dried beans, green vegetables.

❧ CHROMIUM: meat, shellfish, chicken, corn oil, clams, brewer's yeast.

❧ COPPER: chickweed, dried beans, peas, whole wheat, prunes, beef liver, shrimp, most seafood.

❧ IODINE: kelp, onions, seafood.

❧ IRON: Yellow dock, dandelion root, apricots, blackstrap molasses, beets, beet greens, brewer's yeast, chickweed, dulse, egg yolk, grains, sunflower seeds, raisins, prunes, kelp, turnip greens, oats, walnuts, pork liver, beef kidney, beef heart, beef liver, dried peaches, red meat, egg yolks, oysters, beans, asparagus, molasses.

❧ MAGNESIUM: chickweed, dandelion, lemons, grapefruit, figs, yellow corn, nuts, seeds, apples, dark green vegetables.

❧ MANGANESE: chickweed, dandelion, nuts, green leafy vegetables, peas, beets, egg yolks, whole grains, seeds.

❧ PHOSPHORUS: dandelion, oats, meat, poultry, fish, whole grains, eggs, nuts, seeds.

❧ POTASSIUM: dandelion, bananas, cantaloupe, citrus fruits, green leafy vegetables, mint leaves, potatoes, tomatoes, sunflower seeds, watercress.

❧ SELENIUM: whole grains, seafood, seaweed, organ meats, brewer's yeast, garlic, wheat germ, onions, tomatoes, broccoli.

❧ SILICON: chickweed, dandelion, kelp, horsetail.

❧ SULFUR: lean beef, dried beans, fish, eggs, cabbage, garlic, onions.

❧ VANADIUM: fish. (Do not take synthetic supplements of vanadium.)

❧ ZINC: chickweed, round steak, lamb chops, pork loin, wheat germ, brewer's yeast, pumpkin seeds, eggs, nonfat dry milk, ground mustard, oysters.

NUTRITION MISCELLANY

❧ Sugar depletes you of B VITAMINS. The typical American diet contains far too much sugar. Excessive sugar of *any* kind depletes the body of B VITAMINS and minerals, raises cholesterol, overburdens the pancreas, promotes obesity, rotten teeth, parasitic growths (including candida), arthritis, gout, hyperactivity in some, fatigue in others, diabetes, hypoglycemia, and just poor health in general.

🅖 Alcohol depletes you of B VITAMINS and VITAMIN C and interferes with the absorption of CALCIUM.

🅖 If you're going to drink alcohol, take a strong VITAMIN B COMPLEX before, during, and after drinking alcohol. Also drink lots of water. You'll avoid a hangover.

🅖 Antibiotics and vitamin and mineral supplements don't mix too well. Don't take supplements and antibiotics at the same time. Allow at least an hour in between.

🅖 Aspirin triples the excretion rate of VITAMIN C.

🅖 Drugs, even "safe," over-the-counter drugs, induce vitamin deficits. Commonly used cold, allergy, and pain remedies lower VITAMIN A blood levels, the one thing you don't need if you're sick and run-down. VITAMIN A protects mucus membranes of the lungs, throat, and nose against infection; it also protects against infection in general. Diuretics rob you of the VITAMIN B COMPLEX, POTASSIUM, MAGNESIUM, and ZINC. Alcohol depletes you of the B COMPLEX, VITAMIN A, and MAGNESIUM. Triminicol steals VITAMIN C, a potent antibacterial and antiviral vitamin. The list goes on and on.

🅖 A deficiency of VITAMIN A can cause excess excretion of VITAMIN C.

🅖 Oral contraceptives interfere with the body's ability to absorb and utilize VITAMINS B6, B12, C, and FOLIC ACID.

🅖 High protein intake increases the need for VITAMIN B6 (and puts a tremendous strain on your kidneys, especially if you're also taking a diuretic.)

🅖 Most nutrients are absorbed from the small intestine.

🅖 VITAMIN C enhances the utilization of IRON. Take them together.

🅖 Inorganic IRON, such as ferrous sulfate, is not easily assimilated, and it destroys VITAMIN E. If you must use inorganic iron, allow eight hours between taking it and VITAMIN E.

🅖 Large amounts of caffeine block IRON absorption.

🅖 High PHOSPHORUS intake lowers your calcium levels. Main culprits: high meat protein intake and high soft drink intake.

🅖 RNA and DNA supplements should not be taken by gout sufferers, due to a possible increase in uric acid levels.

❧ Strict vegetarians need B12 supplementation.

❧ Excessive use of polyunsaturated fats or oils (meaning, to the total exclusion of saturated fats) can deplete the body of antioxidant VITA-MINS, E, A, D, and K. Some studies even indicate exclusive use of polyunsaturated fats accelerates the aging process. This makes sense: you need ANTIOXIDANTS to get rid of free radicals; free radicals are strongly implicated in the aging process, as well as in many degenerative diseases. Nuts, seeds, grains, whole milk and other dairy products (for the milk tolerant) are good sources of unsaturated and saturated fatty acids.

❧ Synthetic vitamins are made from petroleum products.

❧ Natural VITAMIN E, d-alpha tocopherol (pronounced DEE-alfa toe-KOF-er-ol), d-alpha tocopherylacetate or d-alpha tocopheryl succinate is better absorbed, better utilized, and retained longer in the body than synthetic VITAMIN E. Synthetic VITAMIN E is designated as dl-alpha tocopherol, dl-alpha tocopheryl acetate, or dl-alpha tocopheryl succinate. Note the "L" after the "D." Natural VITAMIN E is much more expensive than synthetic VITAMIN E. Some manufacturers put 90 percent or more of the synthetic variety and only 10 percent or less of the natural VITAMIN E in their products. Because it does contain natural VITAMIN E, they are allowed to call their product (usually in large letters) Natural VITAMIN E. Check the label to see if 1) the contents are of the d-alpha variety only, and/or 2) the manufacturer guarantees the product to be 100 percent natural source. You really do, in this case, get more for your money with the truly natural product.

CAUTION: If you have a rheumatic heart, check with your doctor before taking VITAMIN E for any reason. It can sometimes increase the imbalance between the two sides of the heart caused by rheumatic fever.

❧ Smoking drastically destroys VITAMIN C. Each cigarette "eats up" more than the MDR of VITAMIN C and creates health problems that require even more of this and other vitamins.

❧ Rancid foods destroy VITAMIN E and require additional E to handle the resulting free radicals. Heat destroys VITAMIN E. Some restaurants reheat oil or fat used for french fries and other foods for several days. Rancidity can often result, VITAMIN E is destroyed by the high heat required, and harmful trans fatty acids are produced.

🕷 Chlorinated water destroys VITAMIN E.

🕷 Chlorinated water kills beneficial intestinal flora, including ACI-DOPHILUS.

🕷 Habitual use of laxatives can result in deficiencies of VITAMINS B and C, requiring additional, heavy supplementation. They can also rid you of the beneficial bacteria, ACIDOPHILUS.

🕷 Air and water pollution levels increase the need for ANTIOXIDANTS.

🕷 Emotional stress increases the need for all nutrients.

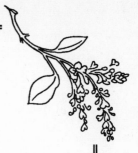

CHAPTER 5

Homeopathy

*Causing a symptom to disappear is very
seldom the cure of any human infirmity.
The true cure is to prevent the symptom.*
                            —Anonymous

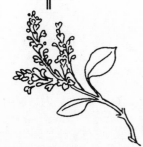

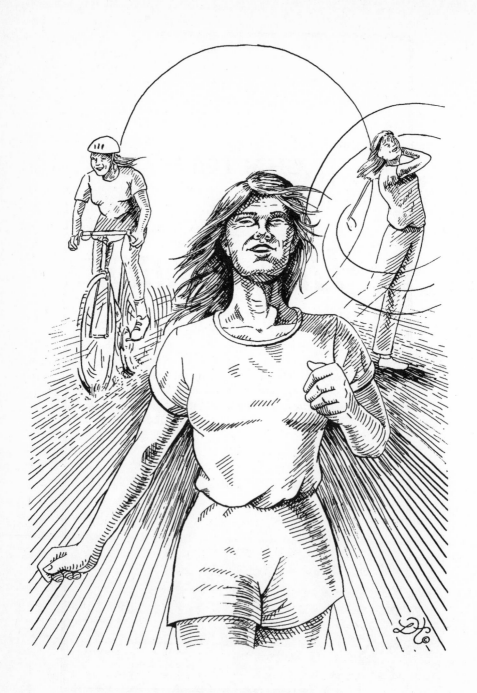

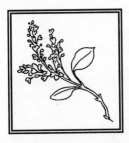

Homeopathy pays more intense attention to physical, mental, and emotional symptoms than any other branch of medicine, yet it does not set about to "cure" symptoms. Instead, homeopathy uses meticulously-garnered symptomatic information from the patient to determine what substance in nature would, if given in overdose, bring about that exact combination of symptoms. (Quinine given in large doses to a healthy person, for instance, produces the symptoms of malaria.) In homeopathy, the symptom-producing substance is administered in minute dilution. Not only do the symptoms then disappear, so does the cause of the imbalance producing those symptoms. The concept is known as the "law of similars." Vaccinations and some allergy treatments work on a related principle.

In contrast to allopathic drugs, homeopathic medicines are given in much smaller doses, and are prescribed to suit a particular individual's personal constitution and array of symptoms, rather than to suit a disease displaying only a certain group of symptoms. Homeopathic remedies are used to prevent illness as well as to treat people who are ill. Notice the difference: homeopathy treats people, not illnesses. A homeopathic doctor will attempt to treat the patient as much on the level of the mind and emotions as on the physical level, believing that all are related to total health. Furthermore, homeopathic medicines are harmless; there are no side effects. Made only from natural substances (mostly plants and minerals), they stimulate the body's own healing abilities, its immune system, to produce a healthy state.

Developed by German physician Samuel Hahnemann, homeopathy became popular in America in the 1800s when its success rate far outstripped "regular" (allopathic) medicine in treating the epidemics of cholera, yellow fever, scarlet fever, and other infectious diseases rampant during that time. Homeopathic hospitals had a death rate of from one-eighth to one-half that of other hospitals.

Founded in 1844, the American Institute of Homeopathy preceded the American Medical Association (A.M.A.) by three years. In fact, one of the A.M.A.'s stated founding purposes was to stem the rising tide of homeopathy! The profession represented by the A.M.A. was in serious danger of being overwhelmed by homeopathy on several fronts, not the least of which was economics. In the early 1900s, 20 to 25 per cent of urban physicians were homeopaths. Not only were more and more people flocking to homeopathic doctors, homeopathy was, and is, an inexpensive form of medicine. Also, homeopathic doctors had graduated from reputable medical schools and could not be dismissed with ridicule on the grounds that they were "snake oil peddlers." (It was also hard to deny that homeopathy worked and caused no harm.[1])

The A.M.A. tried a number of methods to discourage homeopathy, including a rule in their Code of Ethics "excommunicating" any of its physicians from the A.M.A. if they even consulted with a homeopathic doctor, but the method that was eventually most effective was based on the Flexnor Report. This report, published by the Carnegie Foundation in 1910, asserted that standardizing medical training by declaring conventional (allopathic) medical practices and philosophy (the "germ theory") the one and only true and legitimate form of medicine would improve the quality of medical care in America. The A.M.A., the government, and influential funding groups immediately jumped on this bandwagon, setting standards and criteria for medical schools that were biased against any but orthodox, allopathic medicine. The ultimate result of this "improvement" was the "outlawing" of alternative (to allopathic) medicine and the disappearance of all but a few homeopathic medical schools. All black medical schools and a number of women's medical schools also closed their doors.[2]

At the beginning of the twentieth century in the United States, there were over 100 homeopathic hospitals, 1,000 homeopathic pharmacies, and 22 homeopathic medical colleges. Though homeopathy wasn't (and still isn't) illegal, by 1923 only two such colleges remained.

Currently, homeopathy is making a comeback in this country. The importance of stimulating the immune system and treating the whole person is once more being recognized, even by many allopathic doctors. As is

---

1 Kaufman, Martin, *Homeopathy in America*, Bks. Demand, UMI, 1979: Said one allopathic physician at a 1903 A.M.A. meeting, "We must admit that we never fought the homeopath on matters of principles; we fought him because he came into the community and got the business."

2 Ullman, Dana, M.P.H. (Masters in Public Health), *Discovering Homeopathy: Medicine for the 21st. Century*, North Atlantic Books, Berkeley, Ca., 1979.

true for vitamin and mineral therapy, the evidence supporting homeopathy is so overwhelming it can no longer be ignored. There are many recent scientific studies which confirm the efficacy of homeopathy (as well as other alternative medicinal approaches). Europe has always been open to homeopathy and today, depending on the country, anywhere from 20 to nearly 50 per cent of European physicians either prescribe homeopathic medicines or refer patients to homeopaths. This is especially true in Great Britain where the National Health Service pays for homeopathic, as well as allopathic, treatment. The number of homeopathic physicians or other health professionals who use it is growing in America, too.

Homeopathic remedies for non life-threatening problems may be sold over-the-counter in this country, and you'll find many single, and even more combination, homeopathic remedies in health food stores. Single remedies are trickier to use to their highest and best potential because, in homeopathy, symptoms are minutely and distinctly differentiated, and the whole person, not just a set of symptoms, is taken into account. Trial and error with single remedies is possible, though, because homeopathic remedies are both harmless and inexpensive. If you notice no improvement within a few days to a week after beginning a homeopathic remedy, try another. Do not try to combine single remedies to make your own combination; some cancel each other out. (See next chapter for more details.)

Combination remedies—named for the problem they treat—are quite simple to use, though many of them also require close attention to your particular form of ailment. (Are you beginning to see a pattern? Alternative treatments demand and challenge you to pay attention to yourself and to your body.)

For serious illnesses, chronic or acute, you should consult a trained homeopath,[3] but you can safely treat yourself for the more common problems that plague womankind, including the manifestations of menopause. Following are some single homeopathic remedies and some combinations you may find helpful. Although several companies may make a combination for the same condition, the combination name will often be slightly different for each company, so all possible choices will not be listed here. The product inserts will give dosage and instructions. Combination names are italicized, with the company name following in parenthesis.

---

3 For information about homeopathic physicians in your area, call or write the National Center for Homeopathy, 801 North Fairfax Street, Suite 306, Alexandria, VA 22314, (703) 548-7790.

MENOPAUSE IN GENERAL

❧ *MENOPAUSE™* (Nature's Way), for hot flashes, vaginal dryness, insomnia, depression, irritability and other physical and emotional symptoms of menopause. Other companies have similarly-named combinations.

❧ Single remedies—try only one at a time. The best idea would be to consult the *Materia Medica with Repertory*[4] or a homeopathic physician for the subtle nuances of each of these remedies. AMYL NITROSUM, BELLADONNA, BELLIS PERENNIS, CACTUS GRANDIFLORUS. CAULOPHYLLUM, CIMICIFUGA RACEMOSAEX, GELSEMIUM. GLONOINE, IGNATIA, KALI CARBONICUM, KREOSOTUM. LACHESIS, MUREX, NUX MOSCHATA, NUX VOMICA, OOPHORINUM, PULSATILLA, SANGUINARIA, SEPIA, SULPHUR, USTILAGO MAYDIS, ZINCUM VALERIANUM.

ARTHRITIS/JOINT STIFFNESS

Hormonal fluctuations, poor diet, lack of exercise—whatever the cause, many women experience aching joints during the menopausal years. And after, if nothing is done about it. Don't ignore aching joints. They don't usually disappear on their own.

❧ *RHEUMATISM AND MUSCLE FATIGUE™* (Dolisos), for symptomatic relief of acute rheumatic pain, accompanied by muscle fatigue.

❧ Single remedies—try only one at a time: RHUS TOXICODENDRON, ACONITUM NAPELLUS; ARBUTUS ANDRACHNE, SULPHUR, BRYONIA, or ELATERIUM–ECBALIUM.

CONSTIPATION

❧ *CONSTIPATION™* (Dolisos), for temporary relief of occasional bowel irregularity.

❧ SEPIA is good for constipation which seems better after strenuous exercise, crossing legs, and after and before your period.

❧ Other single remedies to try: HYDRASTIS, MAGNESIA MURIATICA, MAGNESIA PHOSPHORICA, IRIS VERSICOLOR.

---

4 Boericke, William, M.D., *Materia Medica with Repertory*, Ninth Edition, Boericke & Tafel, Inc., Santa Rosa, CA., 1927, $29.95.

DEPRESSION, NERVES, IRRITABILITY

❧ *QUIETUDE*™ (Boiron), for stress, tension, insomnia. It helps you adjust to stress, rather than "knocking you out."

❧ *NERVOUSNESS*™ (Boiron), to help you relax without drowsiness.

❧ *RESTLESSNESS*™ (Dolisos), for overexcitement and a general lack of calm.

❧ *NERVOUS IRRITABILITY*™ (Dolisos), for the relief of nervous anticipation generally accompanied by a change of appetite and irritability.

❧ *INSOMNIA AND ANXIETY*™ (Dolisos), for insomnia and anxiety, pure and simple.

❧ *CALM*™ (Dolisos), an aid to calm the feelings of worry, fright, or overexcitement.

❧ *CALMS FORTE*™ (Hylands), for depression with crying jags.

❧ ACONITUM NAPELLUS, for physical and mental restlessness; sleeplessness with tossing and turning and nightmares; and for the after effects of fright. Symptoms worse at night, better after sweating.

❧ ARUM METALLICUM for depression accompanied by recurring thoughts of suicide and feelings of being unloved.

❧ BELLADONNA, for excitability, restlessness and mental hyperactivity. Symptoms better in darkness, quiet, resting, sitting up and worse in light, noise, cold air.

❧ CHAMOMILLA, for hypersensitivity to pain with irritability; inconsolable; sleepiness during the day and insomnia in the evening. Symptoms are relieved by heat and riding in a car and worse when angered.

❧ GELSEMIUM SEMPERVIRENS, for apprehension and exhaustion. Symptoms seem better after urination, sweating, shaking, reclining with head high, but worse after emotionalism, smoking, or when in humid environment.

❧ NUX VOMICA, for irritability, anger, impatience; hyperexcitability and sensitivity; excessive fault finding. Symptoms improve after naps and outbursts, but are worse in early morning, drafts, or after alcohol, coffee, or slight disturbances.

❧ PASSIFLORA INCARNATA, for calming and soothing the nervous system.

✿ SEPIA, for a tendency to depression with feelings of wanting to withdraw from the world and everyone in it; uninterested in sex; irritable. Symptoms seem better after strenuous exercise, crossing legs, and after sleep and worse after getting wet, in cold air, with anger, and before your period.

✿ STRAMONIUM, for anger, irritability with many fears. Symptoms improve with light and warmth, worsen with darkness.

✿ VIBURNUM OPULUS, for excitability and restless sleep. Improvement of symptoms occur with rest, applied pressure, and open air, but worsen before menses, with fright, jarring, or in a closed room.

✿ IGNATIA AMARA, for emotional stress; sighing; nervousness; ill effects of grief. Symptoms seem improved by swallowing, eating, and urination and worse with emotionalism, smoking, touch, and worry.

✿ LACHESIS MUTUS, for irritability. Symptoms are better in the open air and after outbursts, but worse during and after sleep, in warmth and in the sunlight.

EMOTIONS

✿ *MENOPAUSE*™ (Nature's Way), mentioned above, helps stabilize emotions.

✿ *PMS*™ combinations also aid mood swings.

✿ *CALMS FORTE* (Hyland) will calm you down.

✿ CHAMOMILLA, for hypersensitivity to pain with irritability; inconsolable; sleepiness during the day and insomnia in the evening. Symptoms are made better by heat and riding in a car, and worse when angered.

✿ PULSATILLA, for moodiness, sadness with craving for consolation; especially helps the person whose nature is generally changeable, with a tendency to be weepy.

✿ STRAMONIUM, for anger, irritability with many fears; nocturnal fear. Symptoms improve with light and warmth, worsen with darkness.

✿ IGNATIA AMARA, for emotional stress; sighing; nervousness; ill effects of grief. Symptoms seem improved by swallowing, eating, and urination and worse with emotionalism, smoking, touch, and worry.

ENERGY

❧ *FATIGUE*™ (Dolisos), for tiredness resulting from physical strain, insomnia and trauma.

❧ BELLIS PERENNIS—Persistent tiredness.

❧ CALCAREA CARBONICA—Fatigue without cause, muscular weakness, chilliness:

:❧ GELSEMIUM SEMPERVIRENS for exhaustion. Symptoms seem better after urination, sweating, shaking, reclining with head high, but worse after emotionalism, smoking, or when in a humid environment.

ESTROGEN

❧ *GLANDULAR FOR WOMEN*™ (Dolisos), for women's endocrine (glandular) system.

❧ MENOPAUSE combinations.

FIBROIDS

Fibroids are benign tumors which can range in size from small to enormous. Menopause usually "cures" them; that is, after cessation of menstruation, they just disappear. This may not happen, though, for women on ERT. If a fibroid is large enough to cause problems, you may want to try the following.

❧ Single remedies to shrink fibroids; try only one at a time: CALCAREA IODATA, CALCAREA SULPHURICA, KALI HYDRIODICUM, SILICEA.

HAIR

❧ SEPIA for falling hair.

❧ LYCOPODIUM, PHOSPHORICUM ACIDUM, SECALE CORNUTUM-CLAVICEPS PURPUREA, SULPHUR ACIDUM for gray hair. Use only one at a time.

HEADACHE

Fluctuating hormones can be the culprit, here, too. Some women who've had hardly a headache all their lives may experience them now; others may find relief from frequent headaches for the first time in years.

- *HEADACHES/NEURALGIA*™ (Dolisos), for headaches and neuralgia.

- *HEADACHE*™ (Dolisos), for temporary relief of aching at the back of the head, neck or over the eyes.

- BELLADONNA, for bursting headaches. Symptoms better in darkness, quiet, resting, sitting up and worse in light, noise, cold air.

- SEPIA, for headaches whose symptoms seem better after strenuous exercise, crossing legs, and after sleep, and worse after getting wet, in cold air, with anger, and before your period.

- MAGNESIA PHOSPHORICA, for headaches, when symptoms improve with menstrual flow, warmth, pressure, doubling-up; worsen with cold air, night, touch, exhaustion.

- Single remedies: AMYL NITROSUM, CIMICIFUGA RACEMOSAEX, CINCHONA OFFICINALIS, CYPRIPEDIUM, GLONOINE, SANGUINARIA, SEPIA. Try only one at a time.

HEART PALPITATIONS

Though not dangerous, these episodes can be distressing. Often triggered by hot flashes or heavy exercise, they usually pass after a short while. If you experience dizziness, extreme shortness of breath, or pain, however, you should seek professional assistance.

- Single remedies: AMYL NITROSUM, CALCAREA ARSENICA, LACHESIS, SEPIA. Try only one at a time.

HOT FLASHES AND NIGHT SWEATS

- *MENOPAUSE*™ (Nature's Way), for hot flashes.

- SEPIA is good for hot flashes which leave you nauseated, worn out, weak, and depressed.

- LACHESIS MUTUS is another remedy for hot flashes, especially if they seem to originate at the top of your head. Symptoms are better in the open air and after outbursts, but worse before and after sleep, in warmth and in the sunlight.

❧ PULSATILLA for hot flashes whose symptoms occur more when you're indoors, leave you chilled, and wildly emotional.

❧ BELLADONNA will aid flashes that concentrate on your face and you feel irritated and restless; there may be palpitations.

❧ VALERIANA aids hot flashes accompanied by profuse sweating and which are centered on your face.

❧ SANGUINARIA is another remedy for the "face flash," but with this variation, your feet and hands are also flushed with heat.

❧ FERRUM METALLICUM is good for relieving sudden hot flashes and exhaustion.

❧ Other possibilities for hot flashes: AMYL NITROSUM, SANGUINARIA, CIMICIFUGA RACEMOSAIC, ACONITUM NAPELLUS, GLONOINE, IGNATIA, MANGANUM ACETICUM, SULPHUR, SUMBUL, USTILAGO MAYDIS. Use only one at a time.

❧ For night sweats that leave you chilled and irritable, try NUX VOMICA.

❧ SULPHUR is good for night sweats that make you extremely thirsty and heat sensitive.

❧ Other single remedies for night sweats: POPULUS TREMULOIDES, SALVIA, PILOCARPUS MICROPHYLLUS.

❧ For profuse perspiration, try LACHESIS or SEPIA or SULPHURICUM ACIDICUM. The latter is especially useful if the hot flash leaves you trembling and is worse at night and when exercising.

INSOMNIA

❧ *QUIETUDE™* (Boiron), for stress, tension, insomnia. It helps you adjust to stress, rather than "knocking you out."

❧ *INSOMNIA AND ANXIETY™* (Dolisos), for insomnia and anxiety, pure and simple.

❧ ACONITUM NAPELLUS, for physical and mental restlessness; sleeplessness with tossing and turning and nightmares; and for the after effects of fright. Symptoms worse at night, better after sweating.

❧ BELLADONNA, for insomnia, excitability, restlessness and mental hyperactivity.

❧ CHAMOMILLA, for hypersensitivity to pain with irritability; inconsolable; sleepiness during the day and insomnia in the evening. Symptoms better with heat and riding in a car and worse when angered.

❧ PASSIFLORA INCARNATA, for calming and soothing the nervous system; insomnia.

❧ VIBURNUM OPULUS, for restless sleep. Improvement of symptoms occurs with rest, applied pressure, and open air, but worsen before menses, with fright, jarring, or in a closed room.

❧ Other single remedies: ABSINTHIUM; ACONITUM NAPELLUS; ANACARDIUM; ARSENICUM ALBUM; AVENA SATIVA; BELLADONNA; CALCAREA CARBONICA; CAMPHORA; CHAMOMILLA. Try only one at a time.

INVOLUNTARY URINATION

Due to a thinner bladder after menopause, most women experience the occasional minor leaking of urine upon laughing, sneezing, or other activities that put stress on the bladder. If the problem amounts to more than that, you may want to try one of the following.

❧ PULSATILLA for use when you feel insecure about whether you can "hold it" or not. Urination feels imminent almost constantly, though it's not a "full bladder" feeling.

❧ ZINCUM METALLICUM for chronic "dribbles" or slight leakages.

MEMORY

❧ *MENTAL ALERTNESS*™ (Dolisos), for use as an aid to concentration for those who are easily distracted.

❧ Single remedies: AGNUS CASTUS, ANACARDIUM, ARGENTUM NITRICUM, CALCAREA CARBONICA, SELENIUM, SEPIA, SULPHUR, ZINCUM METALLICUM. Try only one at a time.

MENSTRUATION AND PMS

Irregular periods are the regular thing with menopause. Some may be late, some early, some heavy, some light, or there may be a little spotting at ovulation or other times between periods. If you bleed twice as long as usual or spotting continues for 10 or more days, however, it's time to consult with a trusted homeopathic or other health-oriented doctor.

❧ *CYCLEASE™* (Boiron), brings relief from cramping, muscle aches, and soreness.

❧ *MENSTRUAL CRAMPS™* (Dolisos), for treatment of menstrual cramps.

❧ *NATURAL PHASES™* (Boiron), a combination to alleviate many symptoms of PMS, including discomfort, achiness, breast tenderness, bloating, and irritability.

❧ CIMICIFUGA RACEMOSA, for painful menstruation with irritability; exhaustion with oversensitivity to pain and general sick feeling. Symptoms seem better when wrapped warmly, in the open air, and with continuous motion, but are worse with suppressed or delayed periods, alcohol, and/or sitting still.

❧ COLOCYNTHIS, for abdominal, cramping pains generally on left side; spasms. Symptoms improve with hard pressure to area of pain, rest, doubling-up; are worse with emotionalism; anger; before and after urination.

❧ MAGNESIA PHOSPHORICA, for abdominal, cramping pains generally on the right side; headaches; colic. Symptoms improve with menstrual flow, warmth, pressure, doubling-up; worsen with cold air, night, touch, exhaustion.

❧ BORAX, for menses too early; nausea; colic. Symptoms are better around 11 P.M., with pressure, and with cold weather, but are worse with up or down motion and after menses.

❧ LACHESIS MUTUS, for profuse menstruation or "flooding," accompanied by bloating and irritability, even rage. Blood flow is thick and dark. Symptoms are better in the open air and after emotional outbursts, but worse during and after sleep, in warmth, and in the sunlight.

❧ Also good for flooding is SEPIA, especially if periods are close together and there is bloating and a tendency to depression, constipation, headache, backache, and hot flashes. Symptoms seem better after strenuous exercise, crossing legs, and after sleep and worse after getting wet, in cold air, with anger, and right before your period.

❧ NATRUM MURIATICUM, also for flooding with irregular, prolonged periods, tears, exhaustion, headache, water retention, and salt cravings. Symptoms seem better in the open air, after rest, sweating, deep breathing, and irregular meals, but worse between 9 and 11 A.M., in the sun, or in heat.

✷ More flooding help can be had with: IPECACUANHA (bright red continuous flow); BELLADONNA (bright red flow with clots, headaches); SABINA (clotting, intense cramping); SULPHUR (with drenching sweat). Other single remedies useful for heavy bleeding are CHAMOMILLA, TRILLIUM PENDULUM, ARGENTUM METALLICUM, CIMICIFUGA RACEMOSE, PLUMBUM METALLICUM, SEDUM, and USTILAGO MAYDIS. Try only one at a time.

✷ IGNATIA AMARA, for emotional stress; sighing, nervousness, ill effects of grief. Symptoms seem improved by swallowing, eating, and urination and worse with emotionalism, smoking, touch, and worry.

✷ LAC CANINUM, for painful swelling of the breasts. Symptoms seem better in the open air and after cold drinks, but worse for touch, jarring, cold air, wind, and after sleep.

✷ PULSATILLA, for heaviness, achiness in legs before menses. This especially seems to help generally changeable, weepy persons.

SKIN

✷ For liver spots ("age spots"): NATRUM HYPOSULPHURICUM, ARGENTUM NITRICUM, CAULOPHYLLUM, LYCOPODIUM, SEPIA, CARBO ANIMALIS, CORALLIUM. Try only one at a time.

✷ LYCOPODIUM is also good for dry skin.

✷ Additional single remedies for dry skin: ACONITUM NAPELLUS, ARSENICUM ALBUM, BELLADONNA, GRAPHITES, NUX MOSCHATA, PLUMBUM METALLICUM, PSORINUM. Try only one at a time.

VAGINAL DRYNESS

Some see this as a blessing (it makes intercourse painful, so they feel they can now say "no"); others regard it as a curse, cramping their "style." Whatever your case, the following will help eliminate the condition.

✷ *MENOPAUSE*™ (Nature's Way) combination.

✷ *VAGINAL BURNING*™ (Dolisos), for temporary relief of irritation, mild vaginal itching, burning, and chafing.

✷ BELLADONNA for a vagina that is painfully dry and extremely sensitive.

ஃ BRYONIA is useful for those who feel dry all over, including dry stools as well as vagina.

ஃ LYCOPODIUM for dry skin, dry vagina, and dried up self-confidence.

ஃ Other single remedies: ACONITUM NAPELLUS, APIS MELLIFICA, FERRUM PHOSPHORICUM, HYDROPHOBINUM, NATRUM MURIATICUM, SPIRANTHES. Try only one at a time.

VAGINITIS, LEUKORRHEA, CANDIDA

Menopausal women are prone to vaginitis because the hormones that normally maintain the vaginal tissue are reduced. Take the homeopathic remedy you choose one to three times a day for no more than three days or until your symptoms show some change, whichever comes first. Your own system should take over then. If there is no improvement in that time, stop for two days before trying another remedy.

ஃ *YEASTAWAY*™ (Boiron), for getting rid of yeast infections, including Candida albicans. Relieves itching, burning, minor vaginal discharge, and discomfort.

ஃ HYDRASTIS CANADENSIS, for vaginal discharges; itching; cleansing. Symptoms are better with applied pressure, worse with cold, dry air.

ஃ PULSATILLA—discharge is white with consistency of milk or cream, which may or may not be irritating. Discharge flow may increase when you lie down.

ஃ CALCAREA CARBONICA—discharge may be white or yellow and may cause intense itching. Flow may gush off and on.

ஃ GRAPHITES—discharge is thin, white, and burning, gushing forth in large amounts periodically. Back may feel weak, while abdomen may feel tight or tense. Walking increases discharge. Worse in the mornings.

ஃ SEPIA—discharge is yellowish or greenish flow, more profuse when walking and in the mornings. Offensive odor present. May feel pressure in pelvic area. Symptoms worsen between menses or just before them.

ஃ KREOSOTE—Try this remedy first if there is rawness, redness, swelling, soreness, burning, and itching from the discharge. An offensive odor is worse when standing and in the mornings. Symptoms seem better with exposure to heat, hot food, motion, but get worse with exposure to cold, rest, and during menses.

✿ NITRIC ACID—discharge is greenish, brown, flesh-colored, watery, or stringy, acrid and irritating, with an offensive odor; worse after menses.

✿ BORAX—discharge is like white of an egg, or thick and paste-like and may or may not be irritating. There is a sensation of warmth. May be worse between menses. Up or downward motion, as in sitting and rising, may be dreaded. May be sensitive to sudden noises. Symptoms seem better after 11 P.M., with pressure and with cold weather.

✿ More single remedies for vaginitis: ACONITUM NAPELLUS, APIS MELLIFICA, BELLADONNA, CANTHARIS, CROTON TIGLIUM, HELONIAS-CHAMAELIRIUM, HYDRASTIS, SEPIA.

✿ Single remedies for Leukorrhea: CALCAREA CARBONICA, NATRUM MURIATICUM.

VARICOSE VEINS

✿ *VARICOSE VEINS*™ (Dolisos), for relief of varicosis, varicose ailments, and "blood stagnation."

✿ Single remedies: CALCAREA FLUORICA, CARBO VEGETABILIS, CARDUUS MARIANUS, FLUORICUM ACIDUM, HAMAMELIS VIRGINICA, LYCOPODIUM, PULSATILLA, SEPIA, STAPHYSAGRIA, VIPERA, ZINCUM METALLICUM. Try only one at a time.

WEIGHT CONTROL

Thinner women have a more difficult passage through menopause than those with some weight on them. Fat cells produce estrogen.

✿ WEIGHT LOSS™ (Dolisos), for aid in controlling appetite and for conditions of overweight.

✿ Single remedies: AMMONIUM BROMATUM, FUCUS VESICULOSUS, CALCAREA CARBONICA, PHYTOLACCA, THYROID.

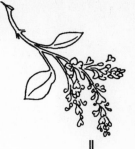

CHAPTER 6

Homeopathy Notebook

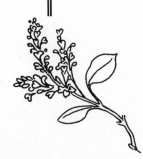

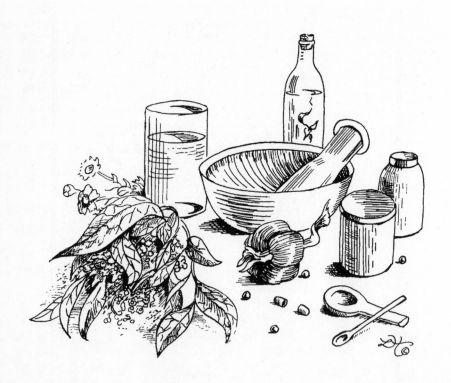

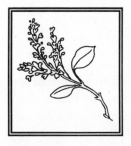 Homeopathic medicines, for best results, should be taken consistently in the ways described below. The medicines come in very small pills or pellets, or liquid formulations. The pills should be allowed to dissolve under the tongue. Liquids should be either placed under the tongue or put in water which is then held in the mouth before swallowing. This will provide the best results.

❧ It is best not to take homeopathic medicines with meals or within 15 to 30 minutes of any food or drink, unless otherwise directed.

❧ It is also best not to brush your teeth within 15 to 30 minutes of taking a homeopathic remedy. Some toothpastes contain mint flavorings, and mint will nullify some remedies.

❧ Try to have your mouth free from any tobacco or flavored substances when you take homeopathic remedies.

❧ In fact, it's best to simply avoid all caffeine, tobacco, and mint while taking homeopathic medicines.

❧ Avoid handling the pills before taking them. Shake them into a spoon or other container and take them from that.

❧ Don't attempt to combine single remedies to make your own homeopathic combination. Some remedies nullify or cancel each other out.

❧ Single remedies are usually taken every 3 to 6 hours for acute conditions. When improvement is definitely observable as being well on the way, you can stop taking the remedy. Your own system should take over from there. If symptoms get worse, continue taking the remedy for a while. They should improve in a day or two. It's known as a "healing crisis" and shows that the remedy is working. Don't go on for days and days or weeks, though. If there is no improvement in a few days to a week, discontinue use of that particular remedy and wait a couple of days before trying another remedy or consult a homeopathic doctor. The remedy will not harm you, but if it isn't helping you, you need to find something that will.

❧ Combination remedies should be taken according to the directions that come with them.

❧ Store homeopathic remedies in a cool, relatively dark place, away from strong smelling substances.

WHERE TO GET HOMEOPATHIC REMEDIES, TAPES, BOOKS, INFORMATION

Your local health food store carries a selection of homeopathic remedies and books. Following are just a few additional sources if your local outlets don't have or can't get what you need. You might check your library for directories of organizations. *New Age Journal* publishes a *Holistic Health Directory* every year ($5.95 in 1992). If you can't find it at a bookstore, you could write them at 342 Western Ave., Brighton, MA 02135.

HAHNEMANN MEDICAL CLINIC
1918 Bonita Ave.
Berkeley, CA 94704
Medical services and ongoing courses in homeopathy.

HAHNEMANN PHARMACY
1918 Bonita Ave.
Berkeley, CA 94704
Homeopathic remedies, kits, tapes, books.

HOMEOPATHIC EDUCATIONAL SERVICES
2124 Kittredge St.
Berkeley, CA 94704
Homeopathic remedies, tapes, kits, books. Send a stamped, self-addressed envelope for a catalog.

NATIONAL CENTER FOR HOMEOPATHY
801 North Fairfax St., Suite 306
Alexandria, VA 22314
(703) 548-7790
Correspondence courses, videos, etc. You can call them for a list of homeopaths in your area.

INTERNATIONAL FOUNDATION FOR HOMEOPATHY
23600 Eastlake Ave. E., #301
Seattle, WA 98102
(206) 324-8230
Sponsors conferences and trains health professionals. They'll also give you a list of homeopaths in your area if you call or write.

AMERICAN INSTITUTE OF HOMEOPATHY
801 North Fairfax St., Suite 306
Alexandria, VA 22314
Organization of homeopathic MDs and dentists. Publishes *Journal of the American Institute of Homeopathy.*

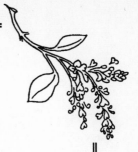

CHAPTER 7

Foods for Menopause

Now learn what and how great benefits a temperate diet will bring along with it. In the first place, you will enjoy good health.

—Horace, 65-8 B.C.

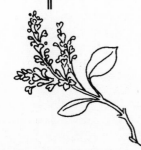

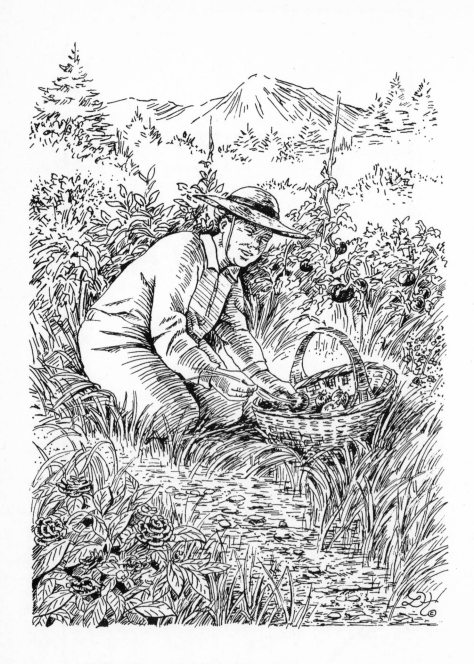

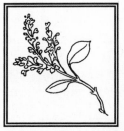

Forget diamonds. Pomegranates and dates may be a girl's best friend. Prescribed since ancient times for women, these two foods contain plant steroids and flavonoids rich in estrogen-precursors, called "PHYTOESTROGENS." Intestinal bacteria transform these compounds into sexual hormones which can then be utilized by the body.

British researchers found that when menopausal women were given foods containing PHYTOESTROGENS (in this case, soy flour and linseed[1]) as 10 percent of their daily calories for two weeks, the level of estrogen in the body increased by 40 percent.[2]

Not that you have to live on pomegranates, dates, soy flour, and linseed. Many of the foods we eat contain PHYTOESTROGENS which can either increase or inhibit estrogen and progesterone levels. Judicious juggling of these foods in your diet can help you have a more mellow menopause.

Other food choices are important, too. It is well known that different categories of foods influence mood and physical status, depending on the neurotransmitters they contain or stimulate your body to produce. A meal heavy in carbohydrates or foods containing the amino acid, tryptophan, for instance, can make you extremely relaxed, even drowsy. If you smoke or imbibe excessive caffeine or alcohol, you automatically place certain constraints on your body and increase the risk of developing certain health problems, not to mention letting a drug dictate how you generally feel from day to day. Your food and lifestyle choices *can* literally determine who you are.

Since you have the power to choose what you will eat and do, you therefore have the power to establish, at the basic, physical level, exactly what and who you will be. Once more, it is brought home to us that only

---

1 Also known as flaxseed.
2 *British Medical Journal*, 301:905, 1990.

we are responsible for our health and bodies; we—not life, nor whim, nor appetite, nor "age," nor doctors or anybody else—*we* are in control. The following information should help you implement your power.

FOODS THAT BOOST OR INHIBIT ESTROGEN

Estrogen Boosters

These foods are useful for the prevention and treatment of menopausal symptoms and osteoporosis. Eat some from this group daily. It is speculated that including these foods (high in phytoestrogens) every day might reduce the risk of developing reproductive-system cancers and heart disease. Pass these foods up most of the time, though, if you are treating breast cancer, PMS, fibroids, ovarian cysts, or other situations that estrogen might exacerbate. In such cases, focus more on the estrogen-inhibiting foods.

animal flesh

dairy foods

eggs

apples, cherries, pomegranates, dates

potatoes

oats and other cereal grains
   (except rye, millet, corn,
buckwheat, white flour, and white rice)

yams

soy beans

eggplant

garlic

tomatoes

carrots

peppers

olives

Estrogen Inhibiting Foods

Concentrate on these foods if you want to reduce your level of estrogen—if, for instance, you are treating PMS, breast cancer, ovarian cysts, or fibroids.

citrus fruits, grapes,
   pineapples, pears, most berries, figs,
   most other fruit (except apples,
   cherries, dates,pomegranates)
cole crops (cabbage, broccoli, etc.)
most vegetables (except the
   estrogen-boosting ones)
immature beans or peas,
   such as green beans

melons

squashes

onions

white rice

white flour

millet

buckwheat

corn

tapioca

ARTHRITIS AND JOINT PROBLEMS

Potato as Villain?

Some people find relief from joint problems by avoiding POTA-TOES, PEPPERS, EGGPLANT, and TOMATOES—all members of the NIGHTSHADE family. To find out if they could be causing you problems, don't eat them for two weeks, then add them back into your diet, one by one. Go slowly and observe carefully. Sometimes a reaction may not occur until several days after you've eaten the particular food. Be sure to read labels, too. You'd be surprised how many items contain tomatoes in some form. Potato starch is another ubiquitous item.

Is Sugar Really Such a Sweet Thing?

Another food that can cause or aggravate arthritis or joint problems for some people is sugar. Try eliminating it from your diet and see what happens.

Vegetable Broth to the Rescue

Having a vegetable broth for lunch, if not for all meals, for several days is often useful for joint problems as well. Cook some celery, green beans, parsley, zucchini, and any other non-starchy vegetable you like in water. Then blend them up and drink them down. This acid-neutralizing broth is high in potassium and aids the body in eliminating toxins. Heavy meat eaters will especially benefit from this regimen frequently.

If you decide to try this over several days, you'll benefit more if you choose days when you can lighten your schedule. It's best to let your body rest as much as possible, using its energy to rid itself of toxins and to heal. Drink plenty of water on these days, too; it will help flush toxins out.

Be aware, also, that as toxins are drawn from tissues and joints where they may have been stored for years, you may not feel too well for a while. Give the body time to do its work, though, and you'll feel better. Having this soup for just one meal a day for an extended time is perfectly fine, providing you have more complete meals the rest of the day.

CAUTION: Do not follow this regimen for every meal for more than three to seven days at a time. It would be OK to do it for a few days several times a year, or even once a month if you wanted to. Detoxing is all well and good, but you can't live on this broth. You need more nutrition than it provides to be healthy. If you do use the broth for all meals several days in a row, don't plunge right back into "normal" eating with, say, a huge seven course meal. The shock to your body could be very damaging. Ease back into your "real" meals gently, gradually. Listen to your body. It wants to be in top shape, and it's wiser than you think.

CONSTIPATION

Constipation is a "disease" of modern, industrial life because we eat too many refined and processed foods (most people think white bread is the best thing since pockets on shirts), we don't drink enough water; we don't exercise enough; we've practically overdosed on antibiotics, we spend a lot of time being stressed-out and uptight (in all respects). Fortunately, knowing the causes, we know the answers.

🍃 ACIDOPHILUS (pronounced ASS-eh-DOFF-ill-us), taken as a liquid (available from some health food stores) at the rate of one tablespoon three times a day or in capsule form, several per meal, will improve digestion in general and colon health in particular. It is a friendly bacteria, normally found in our intestines, that is frequently killed off by antibiotics, either taken for an illness or ingested via commercially-raised meat, or eliminated by a bout of diarrhea. Chlorinated water also kills off acidophilus. Acidophilus is also the bacteria which, under the right conditions, turns milk into yogurt. If you can find a guaranteed live-bacteria yogurt, eating lots of it can be another way to obtain acidophilus. Yogurt is also easy to make yourself. Give it a try for a real taste treat.

🍃 Plenty of FIBER in your diet is necessary for normal elimination. Taking bran, wheat or oat or other grain, or psyllium powder is one way to get it: a tablespoon or two on or in food or in a glass of juice, two or three times a day. You can also use bran as "bread crumbs" for recipes which call for breading or as filler in dishes like meatloaf. A quarter cup of bran in pancakes or biscuits is good, too. CAUTION: Don't take supplements or medication within an hour of taking bran or psyllium. It is indigestible fiber, and if your pills get "stuck" in it, they, too, are likely to pass through your body undigested. When taking bran or psyllium, you *must* drink lots of water!

🍃 Eating four or five servings of fruit and vegetables a day, plus at least two servings of whole grain (bread, cereals, oatmeal, side dishes of brown rice, millet, etc.) is another way. Doing this, you'll obtain VITAMINS and MINERALS, ENZYMES, weight loss, and much pleasant eating, as well as needed fiber. (See Chapter 8 for more on fiber.)

✫ Plenty of LIQUIDS, preferably pure water: 8 to 10 glasses a day also helps eliminate constipation. Hint: Put a two quart bottle or pitcher on your kitchen table or wherever you'll see it all day long. Drink a glass of water every time you pass it. Do not go to bed until that container is empty! If you work outside your home, you might keep a one quart container there and another quart at home. Don't put it in the refrigerator; you won't see it and are apt to forget it. If you want cold water, put ice in it or use an insulated pitcher. Even if you are a person who "never gets thirsty," once you've drunk two quarts of water a day for a few days, you'll begin to want it and find it easy and pleasant to do. Yes, you'll have to go to the bathroom more often, but isn't that what you wanted? Frequent elimination helps move out toxins (and, believe it or not, fat, too!). Also, this much water keeps your skin and other organs hydrated, eliminating and preventing wrinkles, among other things.

✫ EXERCISE is also a must if you want to remove constipation from your life. Exercise, even simply walking ten or fifteen minutes a day, improves all muscle tone, including the muscles necessary to accomplish intestinal peristalsis. Unused muscles atrophy. Intestinal muscles which habitually depend on laxatives, natural or otherwise, grow lazy and need toning.

Exercise helps you relax and handle stress, too. It releases chemicals in your brain that make you feel good, so that, even if all is not necessarily right with the world at the moment, at least you are.

✫ Believe it or not, fat helps, too. It lubricates the mucus lining of the colon. Removing all forms of fat and oils from your diet can be just as harmful as never, or seldom, eating fiber.

HEART

Foreswear Couch Potatohood

People who watched three or more hours of television a day were found in one study to be twice as likely to have elevated cholesterol levels as those who watched considerably less television. The jury is still out on whether this is due to lack of exercise or to consuming high-fat snack foods while watching television.

Avoid Trans Fatty Acids

TRANS FATTY ACIDS are produced when oils are hydrogenated or allowed to become rancid (or both). Hydrogenation is a process which makes liquid oils solid or semi-solid at room temperature. These types of fat are found in margarine, vegetable shortening, and most commercially produced snack foods and desserts. Even though trans fatty acids are unsaturated, it has now been determined that, just like saturated fats, they raise cholesterol levels, leading to increased risk of heart disease. As this risk goes up in postmenopausal women, anyway, it would be wise to avoid trans fatty acids in your diet. It goes without saying that you've already greatly reduced saturated fats, right?

Eat Heart-Healthy Foods

Foods good for your heart are the same ones that improve your overall nutritional status: WHOLE GRAINS, FRESH FRUITS and VEG-ETABLES, LOW-FAT DAIRY products, FISH, skinless POULTRY, NUTS, and SEEDS. All should be of the organic variety, if you can get them. Organic, whole foods may seem more expensive than "regular" super-market foods, but they are much cheaper than drug and doctor bills, and a lot tastier.

HOT FLASHES

Brown is Beautiful

Throw out all white flour and sugar, or anything made from them. Use only whole grain (not the degerminated version) corn meal and corn products. Use only brown, not white rice. Experiment with other whole grains to see if you like rye, buckwheat, millet and barley.

Why? Whole grains contain vitamins and minerals that refining takes away. During menopause you not only need the usual complement of nutrients necessary to function optimally in this hectic society, you need extra, you need every little snippet of nutrition you can lay your hands on, and you can't afford to miss any bets. Your body is undergoing great stress and demanding you supply it with what it needs. If these needs are met, menopause will be a piece of cake. If not, well . . .

As described in the chapter on vitamins, Vitamin E can alleviate hot flashes. Vitamin E just happens to be one of the nutrients strip-mined from grains when they are refined.

You'll probably need more E to put the damper on hot flashes than you'll get from your food, but why fight against yourself and waste your calorie allotment on devitalized food? In addition, no matter how far knowledge of vitamins has come, nutrients naturally occurring in whole foods produce better results in human bodies than taking individual supplements of them. Take supplements, yes, but use them as a support system for good nutrition, not as a substitute.

Curb Caffeine

Caffeine found in coffee, black teas, colas, and chocolate can aggravate hot flashes, probably because, like estrogen depletion itself, it messes with the vasodilation system.

You can wean yourself from coffee, though you may have withdrawal symptoms for a few days. Try switching to herbal teas. There are so many at your local health food store that just trying them out is an adventure. There's an herb tea to suit anybody's taste. Ginseng or yerba maté tea might be a good place to start, if you're trying to kick the coffee habit, and, instead of chocolate, try carob. You can cook with it in powder form, just like cocoa, but since it naturally contains fructose, you can use less sweetening. It's also available in "chocolate chip" form, in tofu- or milk-based drink mixes, and in candies and cookies.

OSTEOPOROSIS

Eat Your Boron

BORON is a trace mineral which aids in the absorption and utilization of CALCIUM. It has also been shown to raise the levels of estrogen in the blood of postmenopausal women by 50 percent. It even began reversing their osteoporosis. Eat that BORON! You'll find it in LEAFY VEGETABLES, NUTS, PEARS, APPLES, and GRAPES. There's even a trace in GRAINS, MEAT, FISH, and DAIRY products. You need only about 3 mg. of BORON a day. Even so, you may have to take a supplement of this mineral to get enough.

And Don't Forget the Calcium

Low-fat or nonfat YOGURT, MILK, and CHEESE are obvious choices when it comes to getting calcium from your foods. Eight ounces of MILK contain about 300 mgs. of calcium, or roughly one-third your daily requirement. Dairy products are problematic for some people, even if they can tolerate lactose. So what then?

No problem. Just add some of the following to your diet every day: SUNFLOWER SEEDS, SESAME SEEDS, TOFU made with calcium chloride (check label), SOYBEANS and soy products, BROCCOLI, CORN TORTILLAS, LEAFY GREENS such as KALE, COLLARD, MUSTARD, or TURNIP GREENS. One cup of KALE contains more calcium than one cup of milk. Even so, most people are not going to eat three cups of kale to get their calcium every day! So, it will probably be necessary for most women to take a calcium supplement of 800 to 1000 mgs. a day, along with MAGNESIUM, VITAMIN D, ZINC, and BORON (all of which aid in CALCIUM's utilization).

A Diet High in Animal Protein Can Cause Calcium Loss

Meat raises the level of phosphorus in the blood and this can leach CALCIUM from your bones if your daily intake of calcium is not enough to balance the phosphorus *and* allow for bone maintenance. Your body will do whatever it has to in order to protect its blood chemistry balance. If it doesn't get it from food, your body will take calcium from your bones to preserve that balance.

You don't have to cut out all meat (though you'd be healthier if you did), just cut down. This is especially important during menopause and beyond, when protecting bone density becomes a primary concern. Combining BEANS (legumes) and WHOLE GRAINS and other vegetables, as well as using LOW-FAT DAIRY products will give you plenty of protein, a more varied diet, and a lower grocery bill. (See Chapter 8 for more on combining vegetables for protein.)

Limit Alcohol and Caffeine

Excessive alcohol intake and heavy coffee drinking are also suspects in the great bone-loss intrigue. Again, the ancient sages had it right: moderation in all things.

Don't Smoke

Smoking is also implicated in bone loss. If you do smoke and want to quit, you might give this old folk remedy a try: mix half a teaspoonful of bicarbonate of soda in a glass of water and drink it two or three times a day. It is speculated that it may reduce withdrawal symptoms by helping to maintain nicotine in the body, allowing it to slowly adjust to doing without nicotine. Another hint: caffeine worsens nicotine-withdrawal symptoms.

Reduce TV Watching

If you watch three to four or more hours of TV a day, you are a couch potato. Couch potatoes, by definition, do not exercise adequately. Lack of exercise leads to lower metabolic rate, poor nutritional status, and bone loss. Just ask an astronaut; NASA instituted exercise routines aboard the shuttle flights to help crew members avoid calcium loss due to inactivity.

WEIGHT LOSS

Sip Soup Slowly, Sally

Researchers at the University of Pennsylvania found that eating soup at the beginning of the meal slows down the process of eating and fills the stomach, thereby giving it time to signal your brain that you are full. You're defeating your purpose if you choose rich, cream-of-something soups, though. They also slow down your eating, of course, but their fat and calorie content makes them less than ideal weight-loss choices. Perhaps you might try the homemade vegetable broth described under "Arthritis."

Following the soup with a large tossed salad with low-fat or no dressing, will further slow your eating and fill you up. A little lemon juice, by the way, makes an excellent dressing for salad.

Simply taking the time to eat slowly will help you to eat less. There is a lag time of about 15 minutes between when a person's stomach is actually full and when a certain chemical is sent to the brain to signal fullness. You could take advantage of this quirk by quitting the table while you still feel a little hungry. Wait 15 minutes and you may have no room for that dessert, after all.

Turn Off the TV and Get Off Your Couch

Maybe one of the simplest ways to lose weight is to cut back on your TV watching. Those who watch three or four or more hours of TV a day not only have higher cholesterol, but also higher weight than less zealous TV watchers. Could be the inactivity; could be too many high-fat snacks; could be both. Come now, couldn't you eliminate at least one half-hour show a day and take a walk instead?

Fork in the Fiber

Fiber fills' em up and moves' em out. Fiber is bulky. It makes you feel full on less. Fiber is chewy; it slows down your eating. It's much more difficult to wolf down a plate of raw vegetables than, say, a Big Mac and an order of fries.

Fiber makes you feel full sooner. Fiber eliminates constipation, moving waste products and toxins and some of the fats you eat quickly through and out of the digestive tract. When you make fiber a part of your daily diet, you feel fuller so you eat less of the fattening foods, you experience less hunger, you're a "regular" gal, you feel better, you lose weight.

Fiber sources: think plants—WHOLE GRAINS, UNPROCESSED OAT and WHEAT or other BRANS, FRUITS, VEGETABLES, SEEDS, including PSYLLIUM SEEDS and HUSKS and FLAXSEED, GUAR GUM, GLUCOMANNEN, even KELP and other SEAWEEDS.

Fling Out Fats

Try to keep your daily total intake of fats of any description (this includes oils) between 10 to 30 grams a day. Many books telling how much fat is in foods are available to help you in this task, and, of course, avoid all trans fatty acids, as previously described.

Foods for Fat Flushing

Flushing out stored fat is aided and abetted if your meals include a small amount of foods containing the amino acid TYRAMINE. This amino acid triggers the release of norepinephrine which tells your body to dissipate fat and flush it out of your system. You need only a small amount with each meal. CAUTION: If you're prone to migraines or are taking antidepressant or blood pressure drugs, tyramine could cause problems. Notice your reactions when you eat these foods.

✸ TYRAMINE-containing foods: AVOCADOS, BANANAS, AGED CHEESES, EGGPLANT, LEMONS, POTATOES, PINEAPPLE, PLUMS, TANGERINES, TOMATOES, and APPLE CIDER VINEGAR. Tips for using apple cider vinegar: Mix 1 or two tablespoons in a glass of water and drink before or after each meal. This will aid digestion, too. Some people like to add a spoonful of honey to the vinegar drink. You can also combine it with an oil and seasonings for a salad dressing. Be sure it is pure apple cider vinegar, not apple cider-flavored vinegar.

Other Fat-fighting Foods

The following foods fight fat through a variety of means. Eat several from this group every day and you'll find the fat just "melting away." No dangerous fad diets or diet pills necessary. Even will power need not be overtaxed.

✸ Foods that fight fat: APPLES, ASPARAGUS (steamed or blanched), BEETS (can dice and add to salads raw, or cook them), CABBAGE (raw or lightly steamed), CARROTS (raw is good), CELERY (raw), CITRUS FRUITS, PECTIN (supplement or from apples), CUCUM-BERS, EGGPLANT (lightly steamed), VEGETABLE OILS (preferably cold pressed, a tablespoon a day), SOYBEANS (well-cooked; can add some to salads), TOMATOES, WATERMELON.

WRINKLES

Smoking promotes wrinkles, eliminating all fat from your diet promotes wrinkles, not drinking six to eight glasses of water (you can count juices and herbal teas) a day promotes wrinkles, not following common sense nutritional guidelines (see Chapter 8) promotes wrinkles, not getting enough VITAMINS A and C and ZINC promotes wrinkles, worrying about getting wrinkles promotes wrinkles, thinking you are over the hill promotes wrinkles.

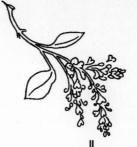

CHAPTER 8

Foods Notebook

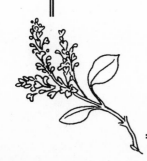

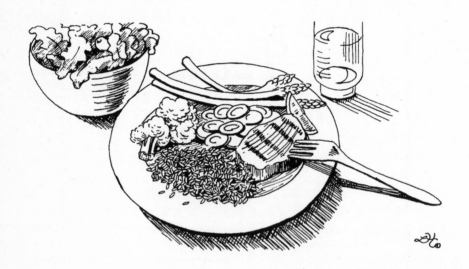

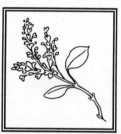

Paying attention to your nutritional needs and following practical health tips can help you trip lightly through the menopause years.

Fact: Menopause increases your nutritional needs to an incredible degree. In some instances (notably calcium), a menopausal woman needs more nutrition than a growing teenager!

Fact: If your adrenal and other glands are not exhausted from a lifetime of poor nutrition, they can pick up some of the slack of hormone production when the ovaries start retiring. The symptoms of adrenal exhaustion include abnormal perspiration, chills, dry mouth, flushing, hypertension, nervousness, tremors—some of the same symptoms attributed to estrogen "deficiency." Well-nourished adrenals can mean an easier menopause.

To better nourish your adrenals and the rest of your body, take your vitamin and mineral supplements and heed the following guidelines.

Eat Plants, Fresh and Natural

This practice will help you to get natural-source vitamins and minerals, and, unless you slather everything in butter and rich sauces, it will automatically provide you with a low-fat, high-fiber diet. This means you should avoid, like the plague, refined carbohydrates (white flour and white sugar), because they are essentially nothing but calories, no matter how "enriched" they claim to be, and they can even rob you of nutrients. Also avoid canned fruits and vegetables, since, obviously, none of these will be fresh—meaning they will have had many of their nutrients destroyed or lost in the processing.

Eat organically grown foods whenever you can. (Organic means grown without chemical fertilizers, insecticides, herbicides, or fungicides.) They contain more nutrients and taste better than conventionally grown foods. As an added bonus, neither their production nor consumption poisons wildlife, the Earth, or you. Organic foods are not widely available (though this is changing rapidly), so do the best you can. Every little bit helps. Persist in requesting them from your local supermarket, and, if you can't have a garden, grow some radishes or lettuce in a flower pot in your kitchen window or plant a tomato in a tub on the patio.

Eat vegetables and fruits raw or lightly steamed, with skins on when feasible. You can even eat many grains "raw" by pouring boiling water over them and letting them sit for several hours. Or use a thermos overnight. They'll still be chewy, but chewable, and absolutely delicious.

Reduce Your Protein Intake, Especially from Meat Sources

Fat and meat have been implicated in many modern-day health problems, but the main reason for reducing meat as source of protein during the menopause and beyond is that it raises the level of phosphorus in the blood, which leaches calcium from the bones. When you do eat meat, remove all visible fat and the skins, and avoid processed and smoked meats (bacon, ham, luncheon meats) and anything else containing nitrates and nitrites. You can use low-fat dairy products as a source of protein, as well as the vegetarian's ploy of combining complementary vegetables (beans and whole grains, for instance) to produce a complete protein comparable to that found in animal sources. (See below.) We humans really don't need as much protein as we've been taught to believe (thanks to the meat and dairy industry, energetic instigators and promoters of the fallacious "Four Food Groups"), and we Americans generally get more than enough, anyway.

Keep Fat Intake Moderate

Even polyunsaturated fats found in vegetable oils are not the innocent angels they were once thought to be. If they've been hydrogenated or partially hydrogenated they contain—or mutate into—trans fatty acids. These are found in margarine, vegetable shortening and other hydrogenated fats and are as nasty about raising cholesterol levels as saturated fats. (Hydrogenation modifies liquid fats so that they become solids or near-solids, making them resistant to spoilage. In the process trans fatty acids are produced.)

What to do? Avoid hydrogenated products. Read the labels. In addition to margarine and vegetable shortening, commercially produced cakes, cookies, doughnuts, pies, puddings, potato chips, and all those other snack foods that are ambrosia to a couch potato's palate are also suspect.

Oxidation (rancidity) of oils also produces trans fatty acids. Fast-food-restaurant french fries are often fried in oil or fat that is reused over several days, oil which becomes rancid, thus producing trans fatty acids and free radicals. Both of these little devils are implicated in the aging process and degenerative diseases.

No, you don't have to avoid all fatty acids (fats and oils); in fact, our bodies must have some in order to function properly. Simply use olive oil or other vegetable oils which remain liquid at room temperature. Even butter, in small amounts, is better for you than hydrogenated oils.

As the ancients have said, moderation is the key in all things. Here's a trick to get butter taste while cutting down on butter usage: Let a pound of butter soften at room temperature. Then, using a food processor, blender, or mixer, blend in about a cup of cold pressed safflower, canola, or other mild-tasting oil. (Oils extracted with a press are better for you than chemically-extracted oils. Fewer nutrients are lost, and no chemical residues contaminate the oil.) The amount of oil to add is a judgment call. It depends on how soft or how solid you want the butter to be when chilled. This trick not only cuts butter intake, it also saves money.

Avoid the Sugar Blues

You can't afford to eat empty calories, and refined sugar contains nothing but calories. Worse than that, it not only gives you nothing, it takes plenty away from you. Refined (white *and* brown, even some "raw") sugar depletes you of B vitamins and the trace mineral chromium, because these nutrients are used up as your body metabolizes refined sugar. (White sugar has all its nutrients refined out of it. The nutrient-rich residue is blackstrap molasses, a very thick, strong-tasting syrup. "Raw" sugar, available from health food stores, is supposedly refined to a lesser degree than white sugar. Some is, some isn't. Some is merely colored and flavored, like the brown sugar commonly used in some baking.) Sugar also raises blood lipid levels in women after menopause, and this in turn contributes to atherosclerosis and heart disease.

If you crave sweets, eat more fruits, taking their phytoestrogen effects into account, and take a chromium picolinate supplement. Chromium normalizes blood sugar, helping to keep the level of sugar at a reasonable level, thereby eliminating sweet-craving. Consider your hormonal level, as well, since an imbalance can sometimes induce sweet cravings. Vitamins, herbs, foods, or other natural means discussed in this book can help you adjust it.

For sweeteners, use raw, unpasteurized honey, stevia herb, malted barley powder, licorice root powder, dried or fresh fruit, unsweetened condensed fruit juice, or fructose. All of these are still sugars, of course, but have the advantage of including at least some nutrients with the sweet taste. They're sweeter than sucrose, so you use less, thereby getting fewer calories, too. They are also utilized differently by our bodies; blood sugar and energy levels are raised, then maintained at an even plateau, before slowly falling off. Refined white cane sugar (sucrose), however, quickly raises your energy level as it rapidly raises your blood-sugar level. Then comes the kicker: It almost as rapidly drops that blood sugar level to below where it was when you first ate the sugar, producing fatigue, drowsiness, depression (sugar "blues") in some and the need for another "hit" of sugar. Does this sound like an addicting, debilitating drug? It is.

Honey is pasturized by the food industry only to keep it from "turning to sugar," i.e., crystalizing. This is for cosmetic purposes only. Crystalization does not harm honey, nor has it spoiled. Honey is antiseptic; it will not support the growth of bacteria or fungus. It will not spoil. It will not even ferment unless it is greatly diluted with water. The high heat of pasturization destroys certain enzymes and nutrients in raw honey. To liquefy crystalized honey: Set the jar in a pan of warm water and heat very slowly and gently over low heat.

Stevia is incredibly sweet; a minute amount goes a long way.

What about aspartame, otherwise known as NutriSweet™ or Equal™? Once again, we are reminded that it's not nice to fool Mother Nature. (For one thing, she's very good at revenge.) Yes, aspartame is composed of naturally occurring amino acids, but it is an unnatural alliance, wrought by Man, not by Nature. Many people have severe allergic reactions to aspartame, and still others are allergic to it without realizing it. Use of aspartame has been linked to headaches, memory loss, dizziness, ringing in the ears, and even seizures in some people.[1] The more you ingest of it, the more likely you are to develop a sensitivity to it. Those who drink a lot of diet soda, to the exclusion of eating healthy foods, are especially at risk. Aspartame alters the amino acid mix in the blood and hence the balance of neurotransmitters in the brain. Once in the body, it is converted to methyl alcohol (a known poison), which is then converted to formaldehyde (a known carcinogen). Lord knows what long-term use of aspartame does to your poor liver, working itself to death trying to detoxify your body of all this. Even (shudder) white sugar is better for you than aspartame.

---

1 Whitaker, Julian Dr., *Health & Healing*, Vol. 3, No. 1, 1/93.

Reduce or Eliminate Salt

Too much salt can cause you to retain water, raise your blood pressure, and is hard on your liver and kidneys. "But, we need salt," many people protest. Well, yes and no, but certainly not in the excess amounts generally ingested by the average American. Common table salt, sodium chloride, is not required as such by the body. Sodium is. And sodium is available right from most of the foods we eat. Many vegetables contain a fair amount of this mineral. Celery, for instance, is quite high in sodium, which is why you'll see it excluded from low-sodium diets.

As far as sodium chloride goes, sun-evaporated sea salt, sold in health food stores, is no better for you than "the leading brand." It contains sodium chloride, i.e., a form of sodium, exactly like other table salt. It does have an advantage over regular table salt, though, because it also contains other minerals naturally occurring in sea water. If you are going to eat salt, anyway, sea salt is better for you, because you at least get other minerals along with your sodium chloride.

Cutting back on or eliminating sodium chloride is neither as difficult nor as horrible as most people think. It's largely a matter of habit-modification and palate-reeducation. Salt substitutes made from herbs and vegetables are delicious, and there are many combinations to choose from. Vegit™, made by Modern Products of Milwaukee, Wisconsin, and found in most health food stores, is one such combination. With no added salt, it contains less than 5 mg. of sodium per serving, yet has a salty taste.

Learning to season with various herbs and spices is another way to do without sodium chloride. It is also fun and enlightening for your tastebuds.

Using no seasoning whatsoever is another route. Once your palate and tastebuds are cleansed of the sodium chloride habit, you'll be delighted and amazed at the wonderful tastes you've been missing. Fresh, organic foods are especially tasty.

And don't worry. You'll still get the sodium your body must have if you eat a variety of vegetables each day, plus almost all processed foods, other people's cooking, and restaurant foods are plenty salty. After a while without salt, this will be abundantly clear to you.

If, after eliminating as much salt as you can, your blood pressure is still too high, try increasing your intake of potassium, found in bananas, oranges, tomatoes, and other foods. The apple cider vinegar drink mentioned earlier is also a good source of potassium.

Can the Caffeine

Caffeine aggravates hot flashes and night sweats, and can make you nervous, besides. Some women find that eliminating coffee, tea, cola, and chocolate not only makes them feel better in general, but may also end problems with cysts in the breasts.

Experiment with the incredible variety of herbal teas. Your taste buds and the rest of your body will be delighted.

Don't Smoke

Smoking causes premature aging and earlier onset of menopause. Nicotine adversely affects the central nervous system. The central nervous system is important in the regulation of hormones, and hormones, as we all know, figure prominently in menopause.

Smoking causes diseases, ill health in general, and lowers your overall nutritional status. If you smoke, you won't feel as well or live as long as nonsmokers.

Furthermore, each and every cigarette a person smokes suspends collagen production for 30–40 minutes. This not only leads to wrinkles, but also slows the healing of injuries. In one study, non-smoking patients with leg-bone surgery recovered a full six months sooner than smokers with the same surgery.

Each cigarette also depletes the smoker of the MDR of vitamin C. Recent information also implicates second-hand smoke. The conclusion is unavoidable: stay away from smoking and from smokers while they are smoking.

Good News!

Improving your nutritional status will make it easier to quit smoking, caffeine, and sugar; quitting smoking, caffeine, and sugar will improve your nutritional status!

FIBER FILLS YOU UP AND FLUSHES YOU OUT!

Types of Fiber

FIBER is the part of plants we cannot break down and convert to other compounds in our digestive systems. It used to be called "roughage," but, whatever it's called, it just goes right through us. There are two kinds of fiber: soluble and insoluble.

SOLUBLE FIBER dissolves in water and is found in some fruits and vegetables, oats and barley, and in beans. (Pectin is a soluble fiber in apples, oranges, peaches and carrots, for example, as well as gums found in oats and beans.)

Soluble fibers lower triglyceride and cholesterol levels, possibly due to their ability to increase the excretion of bile acids made from cholesterol. Oats and oat bran, apples, oranges, berries, peaches, carrots, and beans are useful in this capacity. These foods also appear to improve glucose tolerance by slowing the rate of glucose (sugar) absorption.

INSOLUBLE FIBER will not dissolve in water. Wheat bran, whole grains and vegetables are examples of foods containing it. (Lignin is an insoluble fiber in apples, pears, wheat bran and leafy greens, for instance.) Insoluble fibers like wheat and corn bran absorb water and make stools softer and easier to pass. Therefore, breads and cereals from whole grains (containing the bran—the outer hull—of the grain), plus fruits and vegetables are your best laxatives.

Insoluble fibers also reduce the symptoms of diverticulosis and irritable bowel syndrome. The fiber reduces the transit time of foods in the system, thus lessening irritation. Fiber also appears to protect against colon cancer by speeding transit time and by diluting potential carcinogens.

By filling you up and ushering fats swiftly "down the tube," fiber also helps you loose weight. And, by helping to rid you of old fecal matter you may have been carrying around, fiber not only reduces your weight, it also improves your health by eliminating toxins and improving your ability to absorb nutrients.

So, How Much Fiber Should You Eat?

It is estimated that the average American eats about 11 grams of fiber a day. Recommendations are that we eat at least 30 grams per day. A way to calculate how much fiber you need a day is to multiply your weight by 30 percent. If you weigh 140 pounds, for example, you require 42 grams per day (140 x 0.3).

How Much Do You Eat?

Here is an example of approximately how many grams of fiber some foods contain:

*2 cups brown rice or 1 large baked potato with skin	10-15
*4 slices whole wheat bread	10
*large serving whole grain cereal	5
*1–2 large servings of fruit	5-10
*1–2 servings cooked vegetables	5-10

*½ cup beans, peas, lentils	5
3½ cups air-popped popcorn	4.5
a large sweet potato with skin	4
1 cup prune juice	2.6
½ cup broccoli	2.5
½ cup corn	2
¼ cup raisins	1.5
1 cup raisin bran	8
¾ cup brown rice	3.4
¾ cup white rice	0.7
1 medium to large apple, orange, or pear	4
1 medium to large banana	3

If you ate all of the starred (*) items in one day, you'd have taken in about 45 grams of different types of fiber, and, you would definitely not be hungry.

What About Fiber Supplements?

Different types of fiber serve different purposes, so it's best to get a combination of soluable and insoluable fibers. Most fiber supplements have only one type. Besides, who wants to take a pill when you can have popcorn or a delicious apple?

VEGETABLE COMBINING FOR COMPLETE PROTEINS

Complete protein foods are those which contain all of the eight or nine amino acids it is essential we obtain from our foods because we cannot manufacture them ourselves. These amino acids are called "essential amino acids." Proteins are composed of amino acids. Animal flesh, dairy products, eggs, soybeans, and tofu (made from soybeans) are complete proteins. Other foods contain differing mixtures of the essential amino acids, but not all of them. Combining food 1, containing amino acids a, b, c, and d with food 2, containing complementary amino acids e, f, g, and h will produce a complete protein.

Here's how:
Beans + whole grains (about half and half)
Beans + dairy products (more beans than dairy)
Whole grains + dairy (more grain than dairy)
Eggs, dairy products, and soybeans are complete in themselves
and can therefore complement both beans and grains.

Beans referred to here are mature (not green) beans or peas. Also, beans and peas belong to a family of vegetables known as legumes. Peanuts are a member of this family, too, so peanut butter is not a complete protein by itself. Combine it with whole grain bread, though, and you've got a winner.

Strict vegetarians who eat solely from combination group one, above, must be careful to get enough of vitamin B12, since it's found most abundantly in animal products. It can be done, but requires knowledge and persistence.

MISCELLANY

✍ Acidic beverages (beer, soft drinks, acidic fruit juices) dissolve aluminum. Aluminum is suspected as a culprit in Alzheimer's disease.

✍ Always thoroughly wash raw vegetables and fruits.

✍ Peas contain an antifertility chemical (m-xylohydroquinone[2]).

---

2 Waldron, Maggie, *Cold Spaghetti at Midnight*, Morrow, N.Y. 1992.

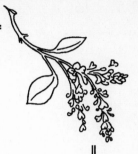

CHAPTER 9

Yoga for Menopause

We are what we say we are. We are self-fulfilling prophecies.

—Anonymous

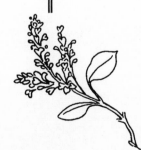

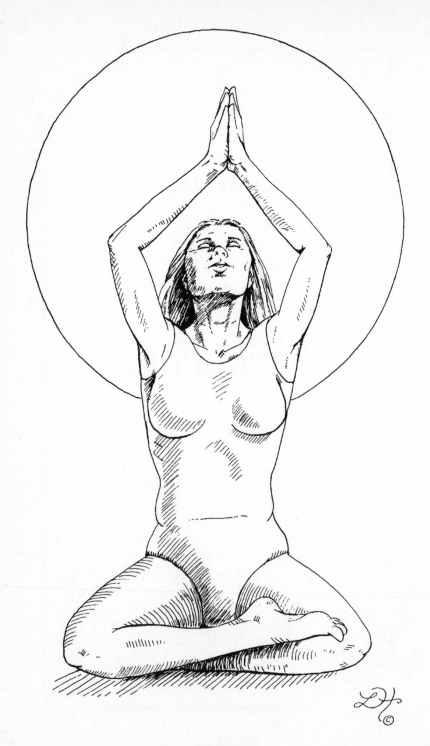

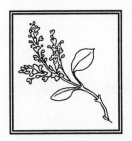

Yoga is a Sanskrit word meaning "union." The ancients of India observed that the various parts of the human being—body, emotions, mind, and spirit—tended to pull a person in four directions at once, often creating unbearable tensions and, hence, dis-ease. For a person to become an integrated whole requires the unification of these disparate parts. This observation was the genesis of yoga, a system of self-development toward integration, perfected by gurus over many centuries.

Several types of yoga exist, each a slightly different approach toward the goal of unity. The one generally thought of when yoga is mentioned in the West is Hatha Yoga, or physical yoga. The postures or poses (*asanas* in Sanskrit) of Hatha Yoga are designed to promote an individual's natural health, beauty, and realization of one's inner power. As such, yoga is not strictly a form of physical exercise, at least not the kind we're normally exhorted to perform. Yoga works gently with the body's own energies and wishes, never forcing anything that would produce and release toxins into the system. With Hatha Yoga you are encouraged to contemplate and focus on poise, balance, beauty, and inner listening as you perform the asanas, never on blood, sweat, tears, and pain.

Anyone of any age or physical ability may safely perform Hatha Yoga postures. You work only to the point your ability allows, never forcing yourself beyond it. Yet with only a few minute's daily practice, you do progress. The secret lies in proper breathing and in holding a pose for a few seconds after you've reached your "limit."

The healing effects of the yoga postures are enhanced if you visualize positive results as you do them. Seeing distressed areas of your body being flooded with increased blood circulation and thus with extra oxygen and with physical massage is extremely beneficial, as does seeing the self you're aiming for. Even if you're stiff as Dorothy's Tin Man when you begin, see yourself performing the movements with suppleness and grace. See yourself flexible, energetic, beautiful, and healthy. (Remember, your body cannot tell the difference between a real and a vividly imagined event. Hypnotized persons can raise blisters on their arms when touched with a pencil eraser they *think* is a lighted match.)

Spending, or we should say, investing ten to fifteen minutes in yoga practice a day will improve your muscle tone, digestion, circulation, respiration, and increase oxygen nourishment of the brain and nerves. In many respects it is like meditation in its effects. Yoga lowers blood pressure in hypertensives; decreases heart rate; improves oxygen utilization in the body, even though, by reducing the respiration rate, oxygen intake is decreased; and induces the alpha brain wave state. Also, like meditation, it slows, and some say, to some extent, reverses the aging process. The gurus say yoga stimulates your life force and thus the body's ability to balance and to heal itself.

As with meditation, other benefits you'll derive from yoga are incalculable and difficult to describe. Healthy, supple, serene, and confident, you'll stride through the world with cares washing over you like waves around the ankles of a giant; you'll know your stressors are there, you'll still have to deal with them, but they will no longer knock you off your course.

Listed below are some common problems associated with menopause and yoga postures that help them. Yoga massages—not jars—the internal organs, nourishing them with increased blood circulation, as well as toning the interior and exterior muscles. Choose one or more of the poses from the category you need to work on, or do them all, as you wish. Just be consistent. Descriptions of how to do the postures are in the Yoga Workbook, next chapter. The postures are cited in alphabetical order, but most routines begin with standing poses, go to the sitting poses, and end with the lying-down postures. A good procedure is to begin each session with the Complete Breath and end with the Corpse Pose, whether they're listed for a particular category or not. Don't give up on a posture as impossible for you. Keep at it and, though the progress may be slow, you will progress. Never force your body, though; never cause pain.

The postures are not to be considered quick-fix remedies, to be done once or twice expecting an immediate cure. Natural remedies work gently with the body, over time. Yoga will most benefit you if you make it part of your daily routine from now on. The *asanas* you practice throughout your life may change as you work on different aspects of yourself. Working out a basic routine to do every day in addition to postures selected to aid a particular problem is an excellent approach.

How to do the postures, general guidelines for practicing yoga, and sample routines are given in the next chapter. It is a good idea to check with your health care provider before beginning any exercise program.

ARTHRITIS, RHEUMATISM

Back Stretch, Bow, Cobra, Fish, Grip, Knee to Chest, Mountain, Posterior Stretch, Shoulder Roll, Shoulder Stand, Circles.

CONSTIPATION

Bow, Corpse Pose, Fish, Knee to Chest, Plow, Posterior Stretch, Uddiyana, Yoga Mudra.

DEPRESSION, NERVES, TENSION

Alternate Nostril Breathing, Complete Breath, Corpse Pose, Mountain, Plow, Shoulder Stand, Sun Salutation, Yoga Mudra.

ENERGY

Complete Breath, Corpse Pose, Shoulder Roll, Yoga Mudra.

HAIR

Scalp Stimulator, Modified Head Stand.

HEADACHE

Corpse Pose, Eye Exercise, Neck Exercise, Plow, Shoulder Roll.

HEART

Shoulder Stand, Sun Salutation.

INSOMNIA

Cobra, Corpse Pose, Locust, Mountain, Posterior Stretch, Shoulder Stand.

MEMORY

Corpse Pose, Modified Head Stand, Shoulder Stand, Sun Salutation.

MENSTRUAL REGULATION

Bow, Cobra, Fish, Locust, Plow, Posterior Stretch, Shoulder Stand, Uddiyana.

OSTEOPOROSIS

Mountain, Sun Salutation.

REPRODUCTIVE ORGANS

Bow, Cobra, Complete Breath, Kneeling Pose, Locust, Posterior Stretch, Uddiyana.

SEX

Complete Breath, Kneeling Pose, Plow, Posterior Stretch, Shoulder Stand, Uddiyana.

SKIN

Including against wrinkles: Lion, Modified Head Stand, Sun Salutation, Posterior Stretch, Shoulder Stand, Yoga Mudra.

VARICOSE VEINS

Shoulder Stand, Sun Salutation.

WEIGHT REGULATION

Bow, Cobra, Fish, Leg Overs, Locust, Plow, Posterior Stretch, Shoulder Stand, Side Raise, Side Stretch, Sun Salutation, Thigh Stretch, Uddiyana, Circles, Yoga Mudra.

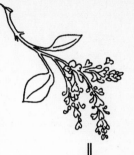

CHAPTER 10

Yoga Notebook & Journal

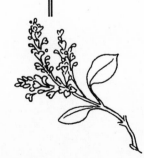

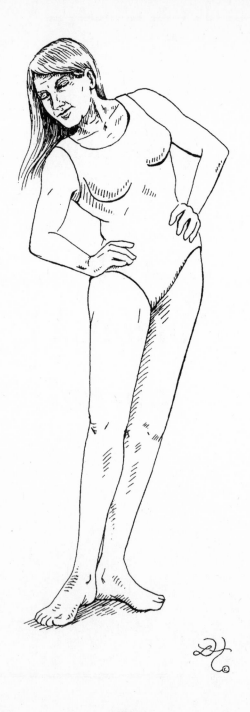

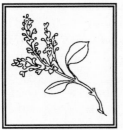

Practicing yoga correctly and comfortably is important in achieving maximum benefits for your efforts. Choose a place where you have plenty of room to stretch out, and you can be assured of twenty or thirty quiet, uninterrupted minutes. The surface should be flat and firm, such as a floor or the warm Earth.

Wear clothing that allows you to move fully and freely. If you can arrange the appropriate conditions, no clothing at all is also good.

Obtain a pad, mat, blanket, or large towel, plus a small pillow to be used only for your yoga practice.

Any time of day is suitable for yoga, though it's best to wait at least an hour and a half after eating before practicing. Most people are more flexible in the afternoons. Some people find that yoga is so invigorating that if they do it in the evenings, they're too awake to sleep. You'll have to find what works best for you, but the efforts you make to do yoga daily will pay big dividends in your quality of life and are well worth it.

Hold each position for a slow count of 10 or more, say, 30, tops. Repeat each pose three or more times, as you are able, or for as many times as seems right for you. Don't overdo, though, trying to set all-time records or something. We're going for quality, here, not quantity.

Take a moment before beginning each session to calm your body and your mind. Sit quietly, breathe slowly, relax your muscles, become serene, letting go all thoughts, worries, and cares. Tell them you will get back to them later, if they are so rude as to be insistent, but that for now you wish to let them go. As you practice the postures, focus on the results you want to accomplish. See them as already accomplished. Pay attention to your body and what it tells you. You may even have a dialogue with a troublesome part to find out what is wrong and what it needs. ("Back, why are you so painful? What can I do to help you?" Maybe it just needs attention and for you to take better care of it. Maybe it would like a new chair for

Also pay attention to each and every movement as you do it. Think of your yoga routine as a choreographed, slow-motion dance. Never make quick, jerky movements. Make every motion graceful and beautiful. See yourself as poised, beautiful, and graceful, like a ballerina. As you visualize and as you do, so shall you become.

SOME YOGA POSES

Notice the word "poses" is often used for the yoga exercises. Yoga is not vigorous, kinetic jumping jacks. You move gently to a position and hold it for a few seconds, thus "striking a pose." You move slowly, focusing your attention on the movement. Yoga is as much a mental activity as it is a physical one.

A rule of thumb in setting up a yoga routine is to balance a forward-bending pose with a backward-bending one and a left-side stretch with a right-side one. Also, generally, as you bend or contract your body, you exhale; as you unbend or expand your body, you inhale. It is very important to follow this breathing rule. And, remember, never force or strain.

&. ALTERNATE NOSTRIL BREATHING—great for energizing.
1. Sit cross-legged on the floor, hands on knees or thighs. Relax, but keep your spine straight. Close your eyes.
2. Position your right hand over your nose, placing the thumb on one side, fingers two and three lightly touching the forehead between the eyebrows, and fingers four and five resting on the side of the nose opposite the thumb.
3. Exhale slowly through both nostrils.
4. Close nostril on thumb, or right, side.
5. Inhale through left nostril for count of 8. (Each of the following is done for 8 counts.)
6. Close left nostril and hold breath. (Both sides now closed.)
7. Open right nostril and exhale.
8. Inhale through right nostril.
9. Close right nostril and hold.
10. Open left nostril and exhale.

This completes one round. Do five rounds. Count slowly and rhythmically, breathing deeply and quietly. After the five rounds, lower your hand to your thigh or knee and continue to sit still with eyes closed for a few moments—an opportune time to meditate.

❧ BACK STRETCH—Sit with your back straight and your legs stretched out before you. Rest your hands on your thighs. Raise your arms slowly over your head and continue in one graceful movement a few inches beyond, leaning your body backwards. Now, keeping your arms outstretched, bring them and your body slowly forward. Bring your hands down to your knees. Relax your neck and let your head bend forward. Hold your knees, bend your elbows outward, aim your forehead at your knees, and pull your body down as far as it is comfortable for you to do so. Keep your knees straight. Hold the position for a count of 20. Slowly straighten up, sliding your hands back up your thighs. Repeat three times. In subsequent practice sessions, move your hands farther down your legs, bit by bit, until you're able to grasp your ankles, then, ultimately, your feet. Don't push yourself, though. Take your time. There is no hurry. There is no contest.

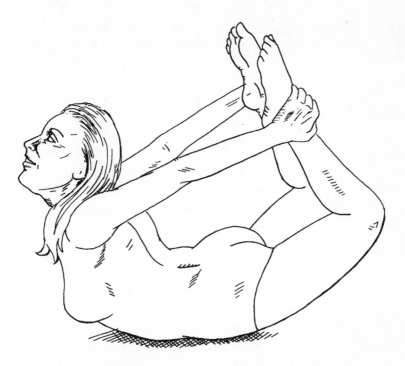

❧ BOW—Lie on your stomach; reach back and grasp your ankles. Inhale. Hold the breath. Raise your legs, chest, head, and legs and arch your back as if you were a bow, waiting for an arrow. Repeat several times, as you are able. CAUTION: The Bow is not recommended for anyone with a peptic ulcer, hernia, or glandular disorders.

❧ CIRCLES—Stand comfortably with your heels touching and your hands on your hips. Bend forward slightly and hold for a count of 5. Now roll and twist from the waist with an exaggerated motion to the left, bending only slightly. Don't bend your knees. Always move slowly. Hold for 5. Again, with exaggerated motion, roll and twist to the back, bending backward slightly. Hold. Now to the right and hold. Move now to the front, but bending slightly lower this time. Repeat all the movements at the new level, holding for five counts in each position. Do the whole routine for a third time at an even lower level. Remember to really exaggerate the roll and twist movements and to hold still for five counts in each position. Move slowly. After the third revolution, straighten up, let your arms hang down by your sides, and relax.

❧ COBRA—Lie on your stomach. Place your hands, palms to the floor, under your shoulders. Inhale. Push up with your arms, raising your chest and head. Hold your head up and back as far as is comfortable. Look up. Your back is arched, but keep your navel touching the floor. Hold for a slow count of 10 or more, still holding your breath. Tell yourself you are as flexible as a cobra. Now exhale as you slowly lower yourself to the floor. Completely relax. Repeat as you wish.

CAUTION: The Cobra is not recommended for anyone with a peptic ulcer, hernia, or glandular disorders.

❧ COMPLETE BREATH (also known as ABDOMINAL BREATHING)—Lie on your back or stand up straight. To first get the hang of it, place your hands with fingertips just touching on your abdomen.

Inhale through your nose and expand only the abdomen. Your fingertips should move apart. Hold a moment, then exhale. Your fingertips
should meet again. Do this slowly, five or ten times.

Now move your hands up to your rib cage. Inhale, expanding only
the rib cage this time. This expands the diaphragm. Again, the fingertips should part as you inhale and then meet as you exhale. Do this several times, slowly.

Place your hands now on your collarbone and raise and lower
your upper chest only, as you inhale and exhale slowly several times.
This is the shallow type of breathing that most of us use most of the
time. Notice the difference?

Now we put these all together for the Complete Breath you've all
been waiting for: Place your hands comfortably at your sides. Relax.
Inhale slowly, expanding in turn your abdomen, diaphragm, and chest,
like a gentle, undulating wave. Hold it a second or two. Now slowly
exhale in the same sequence: abdomen, diaphragm, chest. Notice how
you feel. Repeat several times. This type of breathing has the ability to
calm you and energize you at the same time.

Try to breathe this way all the time. Pause to do it several times a
day, especially when you feel tired or uptight, until it becomes a habit.
This one exercise alone could change your life!

✣ CORPSE POSE—Lie on your back with your arms by your sides,
palms up. Your feet should be slightly apart. Do several Complete
Breaths, concentrating on a soothing wave of relaxation washing over
your body, pushing out all tensions. Just breathe deeply and slowly and
let go of all tensions.

As you slowly inhale, tense the muscles of your toes, feet, and
ankles. Hold the breath a moment, then, as you slowly exhale, relax
your toes, feet, and ankles completely.

Inhale slowly and tighten the muscles of your toes, feet, ankles,
calves, knees, and thighs. Hold, exhale slowly, and relax.

Inhale and tighten the muscles of your toes, feet, ankles, calves,
knees, thighs, hips, pelvic area, and abdomen. Hold the breath. Exhale
and relax them all.

Inhale and tighten your toes, feet, ankles, calves, knees, thighs,
hips, pelvic area, abdomen, hands, wrists, arms, shoulders, and chest.
Exhale slowly as you relax the tensed areas.

Inhale and tense all the previously mentioned parts, adding now
the neck, face, eyes, ears, and scalp. Tighten your tongue, wrinkle your
nose, purse your mouth, squinch the eyes, contract the throat—just

tense up your entire body. Hold your breath and notice how it feels to be so tense. Then exhale and let it all go. Relax. Feel as if you're so heavy and limp you couldn't get up if you wanted to. Enjoy the feeling of total relaxation and calm and peace.

✿ EYE EXERCISE—Inhale and squeeze your eyes tightly shut. Hold for a count of 10 or 20. Now open your eyes as wide as saucers and blink rapidly. With your eyes still wide open, roll your eyes in a complete circle, as if following a strange insect circumnavigating your face. Repeat in the opposite direction. Then look up and down and diagonally several times. Next, close your eyes and breathe deeply several times. Visualize and feel healing energy revitalizing your eyes.

✿ FISH—Lie on your back. Then prop yourself up on your forearms and elbows, raising your upper body. Let your head fall back, with the top of it pointing toward the floor. Slowly lower yourself until the top of your head is resting on the floor. Your back is arched. Your weight should now be on your derriere and your head. Let your arms and hands relax, palms up. Release all other tensions. Breathe slowly from your abdomen. Hold for slow count of 30. Then gently and slowly bring your elbows back into position to support your weight, carefully lift your head, and lightly return your body to its original position. Relax.

✿ GRIP—Sitting on your heels or standing, bring your right hand up and over your shoulder toward the shoulder blades. Bring the left hand up behind the back to meet the right hand at the shoulder blades and join the two hands. Hold a few seconds, then reverse the hands and repeat.

✿ KNEE TO CHEST—Lie on your back, inhale, and bring both knees toward your chest. Grasp the knees with your hands and gently rock back and forth on your back. Lower your legs and exhale. Inhale again, bring your right knee to your chest, holding it with your hands, raise your head and touch your knee with your nose. Hold your breath and the pose for a count of 10. Exhale and lower your head just short of the floor. Repeat five times, inhaling as you raise your head and exhaling as you lower it. Now straighten your right leg and slowly return it to the floor. Repeat the procedure with your left leg. Then raise both your knees to your chest again, touching them with your nose while holding the breath. Lower your legs as you exhale. Relax.

❧ KNEELING POSE—Kneel on the floor, keeping your back straight, then lower yourself until you're sitting on your heels. Now spread your heels and allow yourself to slowly settle to the floor. Go slowly and carefully. Stop if there is any discomfort in your knees.

❧ LION—Pretend you are a lion sitting on some grand library's steps. Sit back on your heels. Place your hands on your knees and stretch your fingers out as far as they'll go. Stick out your tongue like a panting dog, but stiffly, tighten your throat muscles, turn your eyes heavenward, back into your head as far as is comfortable. Exhale as thoroughly as you can and say "Ahhhhh." Don't let anyone take your picture. Relax.

❧ LEG OVERS—Lie on your back with your arms outstretched. Relax. Bring your right knee up toward your chest, then straighten your leg up into the air. Bring it as far toward your head as you can without bending the knee. Now, keeping your shoulders on the floor, lower your right leg to the left until your foot touches the floor, again as far toward your head as you can without straining. Keep your knee straight. Hold this pose for a count of 10. Raise your leg back up into the air and then lower it slowly to its original position on the floor. Now do the same thing with your left leg.

❧ LOCUST—Lie on your stomach and rest your chin on the floor. Make fists with your hands and position them under your groin area, like stubby little support poles. Inhale and with the lower back muscles, raise one leg. Hold a few seconds, exhale, lower the leg and relax. Then do the same thing with the other leg. Repeat as you can without straining. WARNING: If you have a hernia or an acute back problem, don't do this pose.

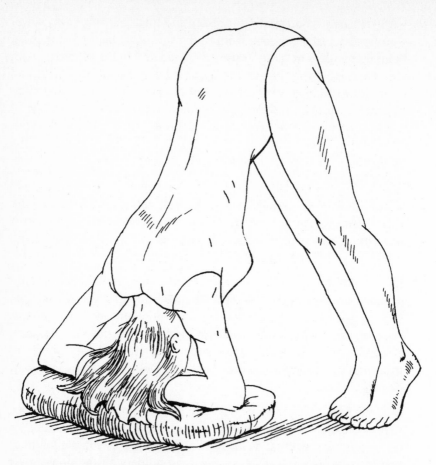

ॐ MODIFIED HEAD STAND—For this posture you'll need a small pillow. A chair pad will do. Kneel and sit on your heels with the pillow six
or eight inches in front of you. Extend your arms and interlace your
fingers. Lean forward and place your clasped hands on the pillow.
Position the top of your head onto the pillow, cradling the back of your
head with your joined hands. The bottom of your toes resting on the
floor, the souls of your feet are now perpendicular to the floor. Pushing your toes against the floor, raise your derriere into the air so that
from the side you look something like an inverted V. Now very slowly
and carefully inch forward with your toes to bring your bent knees up
close to your chest. Your back will be slightly rounded. Hold for a
count of 20. Now lower your knees to the floor and remain in this
position for another count of 20. Slowly raise your head and sit cross-
legged for a few moments, breathing deeply and slowly.

❧ MOUNTAIN—(See illustration on page 148.) Sit cross-legged on the floor. Inhale. Reach both arms up over your head and place hands together as if in prayer. Stretch upward. Breathe as deeply and slowly as you can five or more times. Then, while exhaling, lower your arms. Relax.

❧ NECK EXERCISE—Sit up straight. Nod, or lightly "bounce," your head forward slowly three times. Do the same toward the left shoulder, then to the back, then to the right. Do this three times in each position. Then slowly roll the head all the way around the circuit three times in one direction and three times in the other. This is wonderful to do several times a day to relieve tension which tends to build up in the neck and shoulders.

❧ PLOW—Lie on your back and place your hands under your hips, palms down. Pressing down with your palms, raise your legs up slowly over your body, until your toes touch the floor over your head. Keep the legs straight. Relax your shoulders, arms and hands. Breathe slowly from your abdomen. If necessary, you can rest your knees on your forehead. When you're ready to come out of this posture, inhale and allow your back to be rounded, then simply unroll yourself slowly. Exhale and lie relaxing on the floor for a moment. If you find this position or the shoulder stand uncomfortable during your periods, wait until menstruation is finished before resuming them.

❧ POSTERIOR STRETCH—Sit with legs stretched out straight, then bring your right heel up to your crotch. Inhale, stretch your arms overhead, then hold your breath and bring your arms down toward your left foot. Don't force yourself to reach your foot, go only as far as is comfortable each time. Eventually, you will be able to reach that foot. When you've reached your "limit," hold for a moment and become aware of the stretching muscles. Inch a bit forward if you can. Relax, breathing slowly, while holding this pose for a minute or so. Closing your eyes may help you do this. Inhale and raise yourself gently, stretching your arms once more over your head. Exhale as you lower the arms and relax. Repeat with the other leg and then with both legs. WARNING: Do not try this if you have a slipped disk.

❧ SCALP STIMULATOR—This is one yoga practice that is not done too gently. It should hurt just a little. Grab two fistfuls of hair near the scalp and, by pulling forcefully, rhythmically move the scalp back and forth about 25 times. Release your hair and feel the tingle.

ú SHOULDER ROLL—Relax your shoulders. Pretending you are a loose-jointed rag doll, roll your shoulders forward in a circular motion, four or five times. Repeat, rolling them backwards.

ú SHOULDER STAND—Lie on your back and place your hands under your hips, palms up. Inhale and slowly begin raising your legs and then your trunk, supporting your hips, then your lower back, then your upper back with your hands as you do so. Your chin will be touching your chest, and your body and legs will be straight up in the air. Breathe slowly and hold this pose as long as you wish, but no longer than 15 minutes. When finished, allow your back to "roll out" gently, supporting it with your hands. Once your back is flat, slowly and evenly lower your legs. Relax and lie quietly for a moment. WARNING: This posture is not recommended for those with high blood pressure or an enlarged liver or spleen. (Also see Plow position, p. 162.)

ú SIDE RAISE—Lie on your left side with your left arm bent up at the elbow to support your head. Your right hand is palm down on the floor in front of you. Slowly raise your right leg as far as you can and hold for a count of 5. Lower your leg. Pressing firmly against the floor with your right hand, now raise both your legs a little ways and hold for 5. Keep them together and in line with your body, not letting them sway back or forth. Lower them slowly and then raise them again, this time higher than before. Hold for 5 and lower them. Turn over to your right side and repeat the procedure. Then lie on your back and relax a moment.

ú SIDE STRETCH—Stand with your feet about two feet apart. Slowly and gracefully raise your arms out to the side to shoulder height. Now bend slowly to the left and grasp your left knee.

Your right arm comes over your head to the left. Do not bend the elbow. Do not bend your knees. Hold for a count of 15. Slowly raise yourself upright and repeat the motion to the right. As you become more proficient, you may hold your calf instead of your knee.

✷ THIGH STRETCH—Sit up straight and draw feet in toward your crotch. Put their soles together and hold them firmly. Pull them in toward your body as far as you comfortably can. Slowly lower knees. Hold for a count of 20. Relax, allowing knees to raise. Once more, pull your feet in toward you and lower your knees. Hold. Relax and extend legs.

✷ UDDIYANA (also called ABDOMINAL LIFTS)—Stand with your feet somewhat apart and knees slightly bent, back straight. Place your hands on your thighs with your thumbs up toward your body. (Hands not parallel with legs.) Exhale all the air you can from your lungs and pull in your abdominal muscles. Hold this pose for a second or two. Relax your abdomen, then pull it in again. You are, in effect, "sucking in your gut" and letting it go over and over, without inhaling. Repeat as many times as you can before inhaling. Twenty times on one exhalation is a good number to aim for, over time. This really tightens up the abdominal muscles and massages the abdominal organs. When finished, straighten up, stand comfortably, and breathe deeply and slowly.

✷ YOGA MUDRA—Sit cross-legged, exhale as you lean forward until your forehead touches the floor. Put your arms behind your back and let them rest there, one hand holding the other wrist. Hold as long as you wish, breathing slowly, but not longer than 15 minutes. When finished, inhale and slowly raise yourself back up.

✷ SUN SALUTATION—This is a series of postures that exercises all your muscles and massages your internal organs. It is a moving meditation with which to greet the Sun, both internal and external. Early risers like to literally hail the dawn with the Sun Salutation. The Sun Salutation should be done as a continuous, slow-motion dance, moving gracefully from one posture to the next. The key to remembering when to inhale and exhale is: inhale as you unbend or expand your body, and exhale as you bend or constrict your body.

1. Stand comfortably straight with your feet together. Bring your palms together, as in praying, to your chest. Do this movement slowly, and you can feel yourself becoming poised and composed. This is a wonderful pose all by itself, which you can use anytime to center and calm yourself. Become aware of your body and your Self.

2. Inhale and raise your arms overhead, leaning back slightly. The hands

are apart, no longer touching.

3. Exhale and bend forward, keeping your legs straight. Touch the floor or go as far as you can without straining.

4. Hold the breath. In one graceful movement, bend your left knee and extend your right leg behind you as far as you can, toes on the floor. Place hands on the floor. Tilt your head back and look up.

5. Inhale and hold the breath. Supporting your weight on your hands and right toes, extend your left leg back, parallel to your right leg. Raise your buttocks so that you now form an inverted V. Relax your neck and lower your head between your arms. Exhale and hold. Keep your feet flat on the floor if you can.

6. Continuing to hold the breath, lower your shoulders and knees to the floor, keeping your abdomen in the air a bit.

7. Inhale and gracefully slide into the Cobra position. Hold.

8. Exhaling, raise your rear into the air to make that inverted V again. You are now repeating the positions in reverse order back to position 1.

9. Inhale and repeat position 4, except this time, bring your right leg up and leave the left one back.

10. Exhale and repeat position 3, bending over from waist.

11. Inhaling, repeat position 2, with arms over your head.

12. Exhale and resume position 1, with palms together over your heart.

A FEW SUGGESTED ROUTINES

After a while, you'll want to set up your own daily yoga routine, incorporating those postures useful for a particular difficulty you may be working on. Having two or three routines which you use on succeeding days is a good idea. This way, you can work in more postures without having to spend extra time. Many people like to have a set of postures they consider particularly valuable for themselves to do every day, rotating others throughout the week.

If you are so harried that you think you have no time for yoga some days, at least take the time to do one or two Sun Salutations. Your body, mind, and spirit will be grateful.

&֍ ROUTINE #1. Complete Breath, Side Stretch, Sun Salutation, Knee to Chest, Locust, Corpse Pose.

&֍ ROUTINE #2. Complete Breath, Circles, Back Stretch, Thigh Stretch, Cobra, Corpse Pose.

&֍ ROUTINE #3. Complete Breath, Sun Salutation, Side Stretch, Posterior Stretch, Bow, Yoga Mudra, Alternate Nostril Breathing.

A YOGA JOURNAL

Use this yoga notebook to keep track of your progress and to develop the yoga routines best suited to your needs.

❧

❧

❧

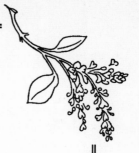

CHAPTER 11

Meditation &
Vizualization

Within each of us, lies the power of our consent to health and to sickness, to riches and to poverty, to freedom and to slavery. It is we who control these and not another.

—Richard Bach
Illusions

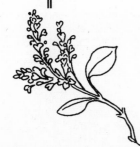

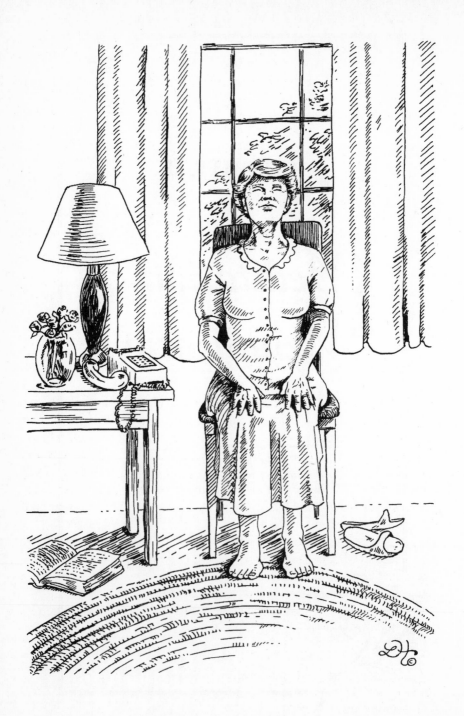

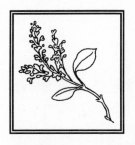

When we learn to *consciously* utilize our own power, we can be free of the role of victim in any circumstance, whether that be victim of "old age," heredity, or of any errant microscopic germ we may encounter. To many, that statement will sound fantastic, naive, idealistic, or just plain stupid. Yet, it is truth.

Isaac Newton would find Einstein's interpretation of gravity and today's quantum physics equally as fantastic. In a way, it is Newton himself who handicaps many Westerners when it comes to accepting the metaphysical (beyond the physical)[1] aspects of mind. He taught—and thousands of Western scientists have taught since—that the world and the universe are nothing but giant machines, big clocks, which, once set in motion, continue unattended, insentient, and unwaveringly forever and ever, amen.

And so, we in the West have had it well drilled into us that we have no real control over our lives, on the one hand, and, conversely, that since all else is insentient, we have God-given superiority and can control anything we want to—given enough technology and power. Collectively and individually, we learn to believe that we are puny nothings and must call in outside experts for any problem, ranging from plumbing, to spiritual guidance, to illness, for only they have the necessary technology and knowledge (power).

This is changing, however, as the new physicists are beginning to realize and accept what Easterners, mystics, and holy persons of all persuasions (including Jesus) have contended for a long time; namely, "There are more things in heaven and earth . . . Than are dreamt of in your philosophy."[2]

There is more to this life and universe than can be physically accounted for, and the power of the human mind is—shall we say it?—unlimited.

---

1 So-called; it may very well turn out to be a physical cause and effect concrete enough to satisfy even Newton. It may be we're just incapable of detecting it yet, much as sixteenth-century scientists knew nothing of radio waves or x-rays.

2 Shakespeare, Wm. *Hamlet,* I, v, 172.

Meditation is a way of beginning to tap into that power—the potential we all have to take control of our bodies and our lives. It is, some have said, a way of tapping into the Infinite.

As a metaphysical journey, meditation, over time, can open all kinds of doors for you; serenity, health, and accessibility to insight and understanding are increased. The mere act of practicing a meditative technique of your choice brings about measurable physiological changes which have been documented repeatedly:

Aging process—slowed
Cholesterol levels—lowered
Pain—reduced or alleviated
Sleep needs—reduced
Cavities—reduced
Brain power—enhanced
Immune system—enhanced
Creativity—boosted
Blood flow to brain—increased by average of 65 percent
Blood pressure—lowered in hypertensives
Ability to cope with stress—enhanced.
Stress hormone levels in blood—lowered.

The list almost sounds like an antidote for menopause! But wait, there's more. As wonderful as all these benefits are, they're only the beginning and may simply be the result of entering a state of passive relaxation (slower breathing, alpha-state brain waves prevalent) once or twice a day. Add visualization and you can begin to take a more active roll in your mental and physical health, tackling specific problems at will.

Dr. O. Carl Simonton and others have had remarkable success working with cancer patients. The patients are taught to meditate and to visualize cancer cells being attacked or eaten by the patient's T-cells or otherwise eliminated from the body. The organ or cancerous portion of the body is visualized (biological accuracy is not required) in its diseased state, the "attack" or elimination is imagined, and then the problem area is seen in the mind's eye as completely healed. Doctors and patients dealing with other problems have also used visualization to favorably affect health.[3]

---

3 Simonton, O. Carl, Matthews-Simonton, Stephanie, and Creighton, James, *Getting Well Again: A Step-by-Step, Self-Help Guide to Overcoming Cancer for Patients and Their Families*, St. Martin's Press, Inc., 1978; Siegel, Bernie S., *Love, Medicine & Miracles*, Harper and Row, New York, 1986.

It works for athletes, too. In a study done with basketball players, the players who practiced in their minds only, visualizing themselves performing perfectly, improved their scoring more than did players who had practiced on the court!

"That's wonderful," you say, "but I'm just going through the menopause, here. And, besides, I can't visualize at all."

Ah ha! Guess what? Meditation and visualization work for hot flashes, too, and you *can* visualize!

Try This

After you read this paragraph, get comfortable, uncross any crossed limbs, close your eyes, take a slow, deep breath and let it out slowly. Think of a lemon. Remember the feel of its yellow, pitted, but smooth skin. Remember its smell, so fresh and clean and lemony as you rub it. Then think of cutting the lemon in half. Hear and feel the knife slice through the lemon and come to rest on the cutting board beneath it. See a drop of the juice clinging to the knife and a drop running down the freshly cut half. See the shiny segments, and smell the suddenly powerful lemon fragrance. Then imagine touching that cut portion of the lemon with your tongue . . .

There. Did your mouth pucker and the saliva flow freely? You have just had a visualization experience. What happened? Your body reacted to an imaginary situation *as if it were real,* and, you have gained an important bit of information and insight you may not have had of before.

Your body cannot tell the difference between a real and an imaginary experience. Isn't that extraordinary? *Your body cannot distinguish between something that you think of vividly and a real experience.* Of course, you're not going to get adequate fluid intake or enough vitamin C to fend off scurvy no matter how often you visualize yourself drinking lemonade. What this simple exercise demonstrates, though, is that *your thoughts influence your body's responses—you, using mental energy alone, can affect your physical reality.*

This is not really that surprising. It happens all the time, but we are mostly unaware of the mind-body connection. Say you hear footsteps approaching your bedroom in the dark of night. If you think it's your spouse returning from a nightly sojourn to the bathroom, no problem. If you live alone—well, your body immediately prepares to save itself and you from harm. You need only think you are in danger for your flight-or-fight mode to kick in, triggering several physiological responses. It is not the outside-of-you physical fact of footsteps in the night that elicits your reaction; it's what you think and *believe* about the footsteps that does it.

Hot Flashes

Now, getting back to hot flashes, try this: Next time you have one or feel one coming on, take a moment and visualize yourself in a very cool, even cold, situation. See yourself standing under a cold shower or cold waterfall, say, in Minnesota in the wintertime, or sitting on a block of ice in a freezer, or rubbing your face with an ice cube, or sliding penguin-like down a glacier—whatever appeals to you or whatever it takes. Try to involve as many of the senses as you can. Remember the lemon exercise? There you employed touch, smell, taste, hearing, and vision. The more senses you can vividly evoke the better. Soon, you'll be able to invoke Antarctica in a split second and won't even have to break stride. You'll be able to visualize a hot flash away, even in mid-sentence. Believe me, this really works.

It works even better if you have time to enter a meditative state before visualizing, but hot flashes seldom give you that chance (though once you get better at it, you may be able to). Other problems are a different story. Regular meditation and visualization (sometimes called guided meditation) can either take care of the situation alone or aid the effectiveness of other therapies. Dr. Simonton and others found that patients using meditation and visualization fared better under traditional treatment and experienced few or none of the side effects normally associated with radiation and chemotherapy. Imagine how well one could do, then, using herbs, vitamins, and other natural therapies with meditation and visualization.

Getting to Alpha—How to Relax

First of all, you need to *relax*. The mind-body connection works both ways. Your mind influences your body, and your body influences your mind. If you relax your body, it's easier to relax your mind.

There are many relaxation techniques. Here's one that works well for me. Like bowling, driving, or meditation, the first few times you try this, you may have to consciously go through the steps, one by one; either mentally or, if you prefer to make a recording for yourself, by listening to a tape. After a little practice you can relax almost instantly, wherever you are.

Find a place where you will not be disturbed. Take the phone off the hook or unplug it. If there are others about, ask that you not be interrupted for half an hour or so. Go where there is a comfortable chair and a door you can close to be alone (without even a cat or a dog). For some people, the bathroom is the only place that qualifies, though its seating accommodations are not usually described as cozy. At any rate, make yourself comfortable, sitting with your feet flat on the floor, your spine (and neck) as straight as is comfortable, and your hands resting easily on your thighs. Do not cross your feet, legs, arms, or hands. Close your eyes.

Sitting is recommended, because you're more likely to drift off to sleep if you do this lying down. For the same reason, it's best to do this before or between meals. You may doze off a few times, anyway, once you get more relaxed than you've probably been in a long time. Don't give up, though. You'll pass through this sleep phase eventually if you keep practicing. While sleep is very renewing and may be just what you need at the moment (hence your "falling" into it once relaxed), it is not the meditative or alpha state (of eight to twelve brain-wave cycles per second) you're aiming for.

OK, here we go. You may want to make a tape of this procedure in a quiet, soothing voice, so you won't have to think about it at first.

A Relaxation Technique

(Begin tape.) Notice the rhythm of your breathing for a few breaths. Let it become slow and regular. Notice how if feels going in and going out. Now a take few deep breaths that are slower than the others. Allow your abdomen (rather than your chest) to expand as you inhale and to subside as you exhale. Then let your breathing seek its own rhythm, continuing, if you can, to breathe from your abdomen.

Now, focus your attention on your feet. Become aware of how they feel, resting on the floor. Relax the muscles of your feet. Focus on your ankles and relax them, too. Then think of the calves of both your legs. Relax those muscles. Just let go; allow them to relax. Now relax your powerful thigh muscles and just let go. Notice how relaxed and heavy your legs and feet are feeling. They are just so relaxed you couldn't move them if you had to.

Now relax your fingers and your thumbs. Next relax your hands and your wrists. Relax your forearms and then your upper arms. You just let go and are so relaxed.

Next relax the muscles of your abdomen. Now your chest. Just let go, You are completely relaxed. Relax your lower back and then your upper back. Let go. Let go. Relax your shoulders. Let them go and just relax. Relax and let go.

Now relax the back of your neck. And the muscles at the back of your head. Relax the muscles over your ears. Relax the top of your head and your forehead. Relax the muscles of your face. Relax your powerful jaw muscles and your throat. Just let go and let your jaw hang slack. Remove your tongue from the roof of your mouth. Relax. You are completely relaxed. And you feel wonderful. Mentally say to yourself, "I am complete-ly relaxed." (End tape.)

You now proceed with meditation, or, if you're not going to meditate at the moment, open your eyes and slowly begin moving. Go on about your day, secure in the knowledge that you can handle anything that comes up.

Use this relaxation technique or a similar one whenever you feel the need to relax, and just before meditation. The process will take only a few minutes at first and can later become almost instantaneous. After a while, you need only say to yourself, "I am completely relaxed." (Or whatever triggering phrase or word you wish). And you will be. All over.

Two More Relaxation Techniques

› After getting comfortable, stare at a point on a wall slightly above eye level for a few seconds. Tell yourself,

"My eyelids are so heavy that I don't think I can keep them open." After a few seconds (they will be getting heavy), close them.

Now, roll your eyeballs up as if to turn them back into your head. Tell yourself again that your eyelids are so heavy that you couldn't open them even if you wanted to. After twenty to thirty seconds (roughly, don't worry about the timing), let your eyeballs relax to their normal position. This simple process will put you quickly into alpha state.

Proceed with the progressive muscle relaxation described above and, thence, into meditation.

› You can do this one anytime you feel yourself getting stressed, no mat-ter where you are—even in the dentist's chair or while driving. Inhale slowly through your nose while mentally counting to four or seven or eight, whatever's comfortable for you. Hold this breath for a count of seven. Exhale through your pursed or slightly-parted lips for a mental count twice your inhalation count. For example, if you inhale for four counts, exhale for eight or more. An inhalation and exhalation is one round. Do several rounds. Then proceed with the progressive muscle relaxation, as above.

Meditation

Now that you are relaxed and may have already entered the alpha state, you are ready to meditate. Meditation is an altered state of con-sciousness, a state of deeply relaxed awareness. You know what is going on around you, but you are not focused on it, and it is not distracting; you are detached. Your brain is not "on hold" or unconscious, but you are not actively thinking. You are passive, as opposed to being actively engaged in thought or action, but you are by no means passive in the sense that others or circumstances can control or influence you without your acquiescence. You are still in control and will be able to respond quickly and normally, should an emergency arise.

The best way to describe meditation might be to say that you quiet your body and your mind so that you can become cognizant or attentive to the deeper portions of your Self—the deeper feelings and wisdom that we all possess, to the peacefulness of unadulterated existence, to the wonder and joy and pure "flabbergastingness" of the peace that truly does "passeth all understanding"—spiritual attunement and awareness.

Achieving and maintaining a meditative state is not easy for most modern Westerners. We have become too accustomed to the eternal chatter of our own stream of consciousness and of our technological toys and tools. Many are uncomfortable with quiet, either external or internal.

Meditation is a skill which can be learned, however, and it is worthwhile to do so. Just like getting to Carnegie Hall, all it takes is practice. Give it ten to twenty minutes, once or twice a day or every other day for a few weeks and you'll be well on your way to being a seasoned meditator. The above-mentioned benefits of meditation are enhanced in long-time meditators.

You already know the first step: total bodily relaxation. That step alone has set you on the road to health. The next step is choosing a method of gently focusing your mind away from its usual chatter and the distractions of daily life.

Four Ways to Meditate

✌ Transcendental Meditation uses the repetition of a *mantra* chosen especially for a student by a teacher or guru. A mantra is a word, often of two syllables, selected for its particular sound vibrations, even when the word is repeated silently. The traditional Sanskrit word used by Eastern yogis and gurus is "Ohm." Try it, out loud or mentally, holding the final "M" like a hum. You can feel it vibrating in your head and your body. Hindus say it is the first sound of the Universe, and they revere its power, much as Christians do The Word.

Apparently any word ending with "M" or "N" can be soothing and healing. Dr. Herbert Benson, author of *The Relaxation Response*,[4] found that his meditating subjects did just fine using the

---

4 Benson, Herbert and Klipper, Miriam Z., Avon Books, N.Y., 1976.

word "one." He had them focus on their breath and mentally say the word every time they exhaled.

If you want to try the mantra method, chose any word or phrase that you like and repeat it, either with the breath or not. Some people like to use "peace," "love," or a Biblical phrase, such as "God is love." Some maintain it is best to use a word with little or no meaning to you, something neutral which will not engender thoughts or extraneous connotations.

Repeat the mantra and focus your attention on it, letting go of any thoughts which come to mind. Don't follow up on them (unless, of course, you think you really did leave the iron plugged in). As they arise—and they will, especially for a beginner—the attention is gently brought back to the mantra, with no mental reprimand or scolding. You simply do it.

After you become more adept at meditating, the mantra will spontaneously fade or disappear after a few minutes, and—wonder of wonders!—no thoughts replace it. (This happens with any method, not just when using a mantra.) Time becomes irrelevant. Your subjective time sense will not tally with the clock time when you've finished your session. You seem suspended in peace and joy. This won't happen in every meditation session, so don't be disappointed if it doesn't. And, don't be disappointed if you blow it the first time it does happen. You may be inclined to think, "I did it!" which, of course, immediately undoes it.

❧ Another method is to focus on the movement of your breath. Become aware of each breath as it enters and leaves your lungs. Keep your attention fixed on the comings and goings of this vital life force (prana in Sanskrit). Its revelations will probably surprise you.

❧ Still another way, the bubble, takes a completely different approach to all those thoughts that want to intrude. You objectively notice a thought as it appears and mentally encapsulate it in a bubble or balloon, like a comic strip character's words. These are very light bubbles and you allow them to float up and out of your consciousness, until no more come and that great suspended silence is achieved. If, for example, the thought that you need to change the oil in the car comes into your mind, you say to yourself as you encase it in a bubble, "Oh, I'm thinking of the car's oil." Then let it go and watch for the next one, until there are no more.

❧ Some people prefer to focus on a mental image to the exclusion of all other thoughts or images. A candle or a mandela is a favorite choice.

You simply gaze steadily at a candle or mandela for two minutes, then close your eyes. Hold the palms of your hands against your eyes for a minute or two while you continue to see the image. Lower your hands. Hold the image in your mind to the exclusion of all other images or thoughts. If you lose the image, literally look for it (with your eyes closed) or open your eyes for a brief look. Then close your eyes and continue.

Whatever method for focusing and quieting your mind you choose, it becomes easier with practice. Soon, you'll have your subconscious trained not to offer superfluous thoughts to try to distract you, for you will have demonstrated your determination not to be distracted. To this end, it is helpful to meditate at the same time and place each session, if at all possible.

Relaxing your body and meditating will bring about physical and psychological benefits in and of themselves. Or, you may take a more active approach and add visualization to your repertoire.

Visualization

As mentioned above, your body and your subconscious does not know the difference between a vividly imagined experience and a real one. You can use this to your advantage in any area of your life, including health and well-being. You must understand, though, that you must "put feet on your prayers" to get the best results. You can visualize yourself as a rich and famous best-selling author all you want, but (at least on this level of existence) nothing will happen until you apply seat of pants to seat of chair and start pounding out those pages. Yes, you still have to eat properly, exercise, and so on to obtain optimum health, but visualization enormously aids and abets the process.

Here's how: Once you reach the meditative or alpha state (you can feel it, almost like a click, over to another "station"), it helps in the beginning to have someone guide you in the following, or similar, steps or to make a tape for yourself and listen to it. The point is to avoid your having to think what to do next, for that would bring you out of the alpha state. After you've done a visualization a couple of times, you won't need an assistant or a tape. Some people won't need one, anyway, but for most it is easier. There are commercially available guided meditation tapes for improving your health, but if you do it yourself, you can tailor it to fit your needs exactly.

Read the following in a calm, soothing voice and be sure to allow several seconds (10 to 60) where a pause is indicated. Read slowly.

A Guided Meditation, a Visualization

(Begin tape.) You are now completely relaxed and at peace. In your mind, see yourself walking across a beautiful, green meadow. It is a pleasantly warm day. Feel the sunlight on your skin and the touch of a gentle breeze. Feel it slightly ruffling your hair. There are wildflowers of many colors growing among the grass. See them, nodding in the breeze. Smell their fragrances and the freshness of a clear, spring day. The earth feels good beneath your feet.

Shortly, you approach a line of trees and begin to hear birds singing and the sound of running water. You know there is a brook just beyond the trees and, walking now beneath the trees, you soon come up on it. It is slightly cooler here, but the sun filters through the leaves and creates intricate patterns on the ground and delicate highlights on the shallow, running water. Hear the water. Hear the birds and feel the coolness and the earth. Reach out and touch the bark of a tree or put your hand into the water. See, feel, hear, and smell everything around you. (Pause.)

Now, you decide to cross the brook, either by taking off your shoes and wading or by using a small bridge you spot a little way downstream. Feel and hear the water or the sound of your feet on wood as you cross the bridge. (Pause.)

Once across the brook, you emerge from the trees and walk across another meadow and up a small knoll. There is a tree of your favorite kind on top of the knoll. You go up to the tree and sit down under it. You feel it against your back and smell its fragrance. You are completely comfortable and at peace. (Pause.)

From your vantage point on the knoll, you look around and give a sigh of contentment. It is all so beautiful and so perfect, this physical body of the Earth. Your thoughts drift to your own physical body. It, too, is in perfect order. You take a moment and see and feel its different parts, internal and external, functioning and working perfectly. Joints move freely and effortlessly. You look at them and move them as if to demonstrate this known fact to yourself. It feels wonderful and you praise them and send them love. You feel admiration and awe at their beautiful intricacy and symmetry. (Pause.) You do this for every part and every function of your body. You see luminous white cells cleansing any areas that may have been lately distressed. (Long pause.)

When you are ready, you arise refreshed and renewed, more in harmony with the Earth and your body than ever before. You walk down the knoll, back across the meadow and the beautiful brook. Once again you walk among the trees and back across the first meadow.

You become aware of the present and of yourself sitting in a chair. Slowly you begin to move a little, and you open your eyes. You feel calm, refreshed, energized, and wonderful. (End tape.)

Additional Comments on the Guided Meditation

Each time you meditate for healing, mentally go first to the same quiet place and then begin your healing visualization. You may, of course, choose your own peaceful setting. It may be by a lake, by the sea, in the mountains, or even in a favorite room or building. Scenes in nature do tend to be the most relaxing, and yet invigorating, though, especially for those who normally get little exposure to them, but *you* are in control. You choose. It doesn't even have to be a place on this planet. It could be on another planet, or someplace completely your own creation.

If you wish, you may focus your healing ministrations only to the areas that are giving you trouble. If you are having heart palpitations, for instance, see your heart working in perfect rhythm. You may want to think of something which operates rhythmically and visualize that (almost as an example for your heart), or see your heart as the object. You could see your heart as a perfect "ticker," for instance, maybe as the gears in a see-through watch, clicking forward in unfailing rhythm. A clock pendulum, pistons of an engine, a musical metronome, or anything that appeals to you would also do the job. These visual similes work very well. The subconscious is computer-like in its literalness and often uses such "puns" in our dreams. Visualizing two or more times a day will optimize the healing process.

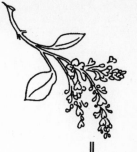

CHAPTER 12

Meditation Journal

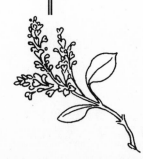

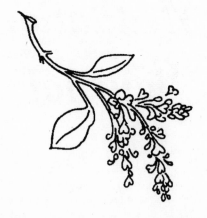

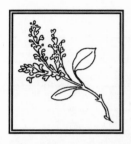 This chapter is provided for you to begin a meditation notebook or journal. Often, insights or understandings will come to you in meditation, and they can be as fleeting as dreams. Life goes on, new insights come, sometimes you forget (conveniently?) a lesson that seemed like a revelation at the time. It is good to be reminded once in a while. A journal can do that for you. The very act of writing can bring new insights. A journal can also be a valuable history of your growth, to treasure for its own sake or, in fallow times, to lift your spirits when you see how far you have come.

🌿 *January*

🌿

❧ *February*

❧

&❧ *March*

&❧ _____

❧ *April*

❧

❧ *May*

❧

❧ *June*

❧

❧ *July*

❧

❧ *August*

❧

❧ *September*

❧

❧ *October*

❧

❧ *November*

❧

❧ *December*

❧

❧

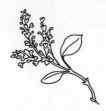

Bibliography

Airola, Paavo. *Every Woman's Book*. Phoenix: Health Plus Publishers, 1979.

Andrecht, Venus Catherine. *The Herb Lady's Notebook: An Outrageous Herbal*. Ramona, CA: Ransom Hill Press, 1992.

Beverly, Cal and Gunden, June, Editors. *New Health Tips Encyclopedia*. Peachtree City, GA: FC & A Publishing, 1992.

Boericke, William, M.D. *Materia Medica with Repertory*, Ninth Edition. Santa Rosa, CA: Boericke & Tafel, Inc., 1927.

Buchman, Dian Dincin. *Herbal Medicine*. New York: Gramercy Publishing Co., 1979.

Carse, Mary. *Herbs of the Earth: A Self-Teaching Guide to Healing Remedies*. Hinesburg, VT: Upper Access Publishers, 1989.

Christopher, John R., with Gileadi, Cathy. *Every Woman's Herbal*. Springville, Utah: Christopher Publications, 1987.

Dunne, Lavon J. and Kirschmann, John D. *Nutrition Almanac*, Third Edition. New York: McGraw-Hill Publishing Co., 1990.

Editors of Rodale Press. *Field Guide to Wild Herbs*. Emmaus, PA: Rodale Press, Inc., 1977.

Fortisevn, Zeke. *Global Herb Manual*. Tofield, Alberta, Canada: Global Health Ltd., 1988.

Hutchens, Alma R. *Indian Herbalogy of North America*. Boston: Shambhala Publications, 1973.

Kadans, Joseph M. *Modern Encyclopedia of Herbs.* West Nyack, NY: Parker Publishing Co., Inc., 1970.

Kilham, Chris. *An Introduction to Homeopathy.* Norwood, PA: Boiron Educational Institute, 1991.

_____. *About Homeopathic Remedies.* Norwood, PA: Boiron Educational Institute, 1991.

Mindell, Earl. *Earl Mindell's Vitamin Bible.* New York: Warner Books, 1985.

Niles, Beth and Casey, Gina. *About Homeopathic Remedies for Women.* Norwood, PA: Boiron Educational Institute, 1992.

Parvati, Jeannine. *Hygieia—A Woman's Herbal.* Berkeley, CA: Freestone Pub. Co., 1978.

Passwater, Richard A. *Super-Nutrition: Megavitamin Revolution,* New York: Pocket Books, 1975.

Rosenberg, Harold and Feldzamen, A. N. *The Book of Vitamin Therapy.* New York: G. P. Putnam's Sons, 1974.

Santillo, Humbart. *Natural Healing with Herbs.* Prescott, AZ: Hohm Press, 1984.

Tierra, Michael. *The Way of Herbs.* New York: Pocket Books, 1980.

Ullman, Dana. *Discovering Homeopathy: Medicine for the 21st Century.* Berkeley, CA: North Atlantic Books, 1979.

Waldron, Maggie. *Cold Spaghetti at Midnight.* New York: Morrow, 1992.

Weed, Susun S. *Wise Woman Herbal: Healing Wise.* Woodstock, NY: Ash Tree Publishing, 1989.

_____. *Wise Woman Ways, Menopausal Years.* Woodstock, NY: Ash Tree Publishing, 1992.

Weiner, Michael. *Weiner's Herbal.* Mill Valley, CA: Quantum Books, 1990.

_____. *The Herbal Healthline,* Vol. 2, Nos. 1, 2, & 3, San Rafael, CA: Advanced Research Press, Inc., 1991.

Weiner, Michael. *Earth Medicine, Earth Food,* Columbine, New York: Fawcett 1972.

Wood, Robert S. *Homeopathy—Medicine That Works!* Pollock Pines, CA: Condor Books, 1990.

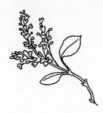

Index

— D —

STAY IN TOUCH

On the following pages you will find listed, with their current prices, some of the books now available on related subjects. Your book dealer stocks most of these and will stock new titles in the Llewellyn series as they become available. We urge your patronage.

To obtain our full catalog, to keep informed about new titles as they are released and to benefit from informative articles and helpful news, you are invited to write for our bi-monthly news magazine/catalog, *Llewellyn's New Worlds of Mind and Spirit*. A sample copy is free, and it will continue coming to you at no cost as long as you are an active mail customer. Or you may subscribe for just $10.00 in U.S.A. and Canada ($20.00 overseas, first class mail). Many bookstores also have New Worlds available to their customers. Ask for it.

Stay in touch! In *New Worlds'* pages you will find news and features about new books, tapes and services, announcements of meetings and seminars, articles helpful to our readers, news of authors, products and services, special money-making opportunities, and much more.

Llewellyn's New Worlds of Mind and Spirit
P.O. Box 64383-K596, St. Paul, MN 55164-0383, U.S.A.
* * *

TO ORDER BOOKS AND TAPES

If your book dealer does not have the books described on the following pages readily available, you may order them direct from the publisher by sending full price in U.S. funds, plus $3.00 for postage and handling for orders *under* $10.00; $4.00 for orders *over* $10.00. There are no postage and handling charges for orders over $50.00. Postage and handling rates are subject to change. UPS Delivery: We ship UPS whenever possible. Delivery guaranteed. Provide your street address as UPS does not deliver to P.O. Boxes. UPS to Canada requires a $50.00 minimum order. Allow 4-6 weeks for delivery. Orders outside the U.S.A. and Canada: Airmail—add retail price of book; add $5.00 for each non-book item (tapes, etc.); add $1.00 per item for surface mail.

FOR GROUP STUDY AND PURCHASE

Because there is a great deal of interest in group discussion and study of the subject matter of this book, we feel that we should encourage the adoption and use of this particular book by such groups by offering a special quantity price to group leaders or agents.

Our Special Quantity Price for a minimum order of five copies of *Secrets of a Natural Menopause* is $44.85 cash-with-order. This price includes postage and handling within the United States. Minnesota residents must add 6.5% sales tax. For additional quantities, please order in multiples of five. For Canadian and foreign orders, add postage and handling charges as above. Credit card (VISA, MasterCard, American Express) orders are accepted. Charge card orders only may be phoned in free within the U.S.A. or Canada by dialing 1-800-THE-MOON. For customer service, call 1-612-291-1970. Mail orders to:

LLEWELLYN PUBLICATIONS
P.O. Box 64383-K596, St. Paul, MN 55164-0383, U.S.A.

Prices subject to change without notice.

THE COMPLETE HANDBOOK OF NATURAL HEALING
by Marcia Starck

Got an itch that won't go away? Want a massage but don't know the difference between Rolfing, Reichian Therapy and Reflexology? Tired of going to the family doctor for minor illnesses that you know you could treat at home—if you just knew how?

Designed to function as a home reference guide (yet enjoyable and interesting enough to be read straight through), this book addresses all natural healing modalities in use today: dietary regimes, nutritional supplements, cleansing and detoxification, vitamins and minerals, herbology, homeopathic medicine and cell salts, traditional Chinese medicine, Ayurvedic medicine, body work therapies, exercise, mental and spiritual therapies, and more. In addition, a section of 41 specific ailments outlines natural treatments for everything from acne to varicose veins.

0-87542-742-1, 416 pgs., 6 x 9 , softcover   **$12.95**

THE HEALER'S MANUAL
A Beginner's Guide to Vibrational Therapies
Ted Andrews

Did you know that a certain Mozart symphony can ease digestion problems ... that swelling often indicates being stuck in outworn patterns ... that breathing pink is good for skin conditions and loneliness? Most disease stems from a metaphysical base. While we are constantly being exposed to viruses and bacteria, it is our unbalanced or blocked emotions, attitudes and thoughts that deplete our natural physical energies and make us more susceptible to "catching a cold" or manifesting some other physical problem.

Healing, as approached in *The Healer's Manual,* involves locating and removing energy blockages wherever they occur—physical or otherwise. This book is an easy guide to simple vibrational healing therapies that anyone can learn to apply to restore homeostasis to their body's energy system. By employing sound, color, fragrance, etheric touch and flower/gem elixers, you can participate actively within the healing of your body and the opening of higher perceptions. You will discover that you can heal more aspects of your life than you ever thought possible.

0-87542-007-9, 256 pgs., 6 x 9, illus., softcover   **$10.00**

THE JOY OF HEALTH
A Doctor's Guide to Nutrition and Alternative Medicine
by Zoltan P. Rona M.D., M.Sc.
Finally, a medical doctor objectively explores the benefits and pitfalls of alternative health care, based on exceptional nutritional scholarship, long clinical practice, and wide-ranging interactions with "established" and alternative practitioners throughout North America.

The Joy of Health is must reading before you seek the advice of an alternative health care provider. Can a chiropractor or naturopath help your condition? What are viable alternatives to standard cancer care? Is Candida a real disease? Can you really extend your life with megavitamins? Might hidden food allergies be the root of many physical and emotional problems?
- Get clear-cut answers to the most commonly asked questions about nutrition and preventive medicine
- Explore various treatments for 47 conditions and diseases
- Make informed choices about food, diets and supplements
- Discover startling information about food allergies and related conditions
- Explore 20 different types of diets and recipes
- Cut through advertising claims and vested-interest scare tactics
- Empower yourself to achieve a high level of wellness

0-87542-684-0, 264 pgs., 6 x 9, softcover   **$12.95**

HEALING THE FEMININE
Reclaiming Woman's Voice (formerly *Reclaiming Woman's Voice*)
by Lesley Irene Shore, Ph.D.
Most self-help books for women inadvertently add to women's difficulties by offering ways to battle symptoms of distress without examining the underlying causes. One of the first of its kind, *Healing the Feminine* chronicles the struggles and triumphs of a psychologist and her clients on their personal journeys to self-discovery and wholeness.

Tracing much of women's distress to society's devaluation of the feminine, Dr. Shore illustrates the need for both men and women to reclaim their hidden but vital feminine aspects. Reconnecting with the feminine entails affirming the female experience, the female body, and the female way of being. Through a variety of methods that include breathing exercises, mental imagery, and living in tune with nature, we can learn to hear our hidden "Woman's Voice" and begin the journey to wholeness and peace.

ISBN: 1-56718-667-X, 5¼ x 8, 208 pp., softcover   **$9.95**

JUDE'S HERBAL HOME REMEDIES
Natural Health, Beauty & Home-Care Secrets
by Jude C. Williams, M.H.

There's a pharmacy—in your spice cabinet! In the course of daily life we all encounter problems that can be easily remedied through the use of common herbs—headaches, dandruff, insomnia, colds, muscle aches, burns—and a host of other afflictions known to humankind. *Jude's Herbal Home Remedies* is a simple guide to self care that will benefit beginning or experienced herbalists with its wealth of practical advice. Most of the herbs listed are easy to obtain.

Discover how cayenne pepper promotes hair growth, why cranberry juice is a good treatment for asthma attacks, how to make a potent juice to flush out fat, how to make your own deodorants and perfumes, what herbs will get fleas off your pet, how to keep cut flowers fresh longer … the remedies and hints go on and on!

This book gives you instructions for teas, salves, tinctures, tonics, poultices, along with addresses for obtaining the herbs. Dangerous and controversial herbs are also discussed.

Grab this book and a cup of herbal tea, and discover from a Master Herbalist more than 800 ways to a simpler, more natural way of life.

0-87542-869-X, 240 pgs., 6 x 9, illus., softcover **$9.95**

TAMING THE DIET DRAGON
Using Language & Imagery for Weight Control and Body Transformation
by Constance C. Kirk

Do you find dieting a struggle? Do you feel deprived, frustrated and hopeless in your failed attempts to reach and maintain your ideal image? The dismally low success rate of only 5 percent for losing fat and maintaining ideal weight is not because the traditional approaches of diet and exercise do not work. It is because the dieter fails to act in consistently positive ways.

This book is about doing something different. *Taming the Diet Dragon* teaches how to end the struggle and pain of diet and exercise, and successfully lose weight and keep it off. It's about changing the way you think, which in turn changes the way you behave, and even changes your physiology and metabolism! It ultimately is about creating your own reality and fulfilling your best potential.

How do you tame the diet dragon? First through imagery, the quickest way to affect perception and physiology. Secondly through language, necessary to effect long-term changes in attitude, faith and belief. And thirdly through experiential skills, useful in focusing on awareness which is beyond words or images.

1-56718-383-2, 256 pgs., illus., mass market **$4.99**

Prices subject to change without notice.

HEALING HERBS & HEALTH FOODS OF THE ZODIAC
by Ada Muir, Introduction by Jude C. Williams, M.H.

There was a time when every doctor was also an astrologer, for a knowledge of astrology was considered essential for diagnosing and curing an illness. *Healing Herbs and Health Foods of the Zodiac* reclaims that ancient healing tradition in a combined reprinting of two Ada Muir books: Healing Herbs of the Zodiac and Health and the Sun Signs: Cell Salts in Medicinal Astrology.

The first part of this book covers the ills most often found in each zodiacal sign, along with the herbs attributed to healing those ills. For example, nosebleeds are associated with Aries, and cayenne pepper is the historical herbal treatment. More than 70 herbs are covered in all, with illustrations of each herb to aid in identification.

The second part of the book covers the special mineral or cell salt needs of each sign. Cell salts, contained in fruits and vegetables, are necessary for the healthy activity of the human body. For example, the cell salt of Libra is sodium phosphate, used to maintain the balance between acids and alkalis. It's found in celery, spinach and figs.

In her introduction, Master Herbalist and author Jude C. Williams increases the practical use of this book by outlining the basics of harvesting herbs and preparing tinctures, salves and teas.

0-87542-575-5, 192 pgs., mass market, illus.   **$3.99**

HOLISTIC AROMATHERAPY
Balance the Body and Soul with Essential Oils
by Ann Berwick

For thousands of years, aromatherapy—the therapeutic use of the essential oils of aromatic plants—has been used for the benefit of mankind. These oils are highly concentrated forms of herbal energy that represent the soul, or life force, of the plant. When the aromatic vapor is inhaled, it can influence areas of the brain inaccessible to conscious control such as emotions and hormonal responses. Application of the oils in massage can enhance the benefits of body work on the muscular, lymphatic and nervous systems. By cutaneous application of the oils, we can influence more deeply the main body systems.

This is the first complete guide to holistic aromatherapy—what it is, how and why it works. Written from the perspective of a practicing aromatherapist, *Holistic Aromatherapy* provides insights into the magic of creating body balance through the use of individually blended oils, and it offers professional secrets of working with these potent substances on the physical, mental, emotional and spiritual levels.

ISBN: 0-87542-033-8, 240 pgs., 6 x 9, illus., softbound   **$12.95**

AWAKENING THE LIFE FORCE
the Philosophy & Psychology of "Spontaneous Yoga"
by Rajarshi Muni

This book is about higher yoga—not physical exercises or meditation to achieve inner peace and happiness (though these may be its by-products or used in preparation for higher yoga). Awakening the Life Force is about a proven process by which you can achieve, eternally, liberation from the limitations of time and space, unlimited divine powers, and an immortal, physically perfect divine body that is retained forever. The sages who composed the ancient scriptures achieved such a state, as have men and women of all religious traditions. How? Through the process of "spontaneous" yoga.

In spontaneous yoga, the body and mind are surrendered to the spontaneous workings of the awakened life force: prana. This awakened prana works in its own amazing way to purify the physical and nonphysical bodies of an individual. Whatever path, religion or teaching you follow, Awakening the Life Force can help you understand the fascinating physical and metaphysical cosmos in which you live. It reveals how anyone with genuine sincerity can practice dharma, or pure conscious living, which results in prosperity, pleasure, happiness, and the joy of selflessness.

0-87542-581-X, 224 pgs., 7 x 10, 8 color plates, softcover **$15.00**

ENERGIZE!
The Alchemy of Breath & Movement for Health & Transformation
by Elrond, Juliana and Sophia Blawyn and Suzanne Jones

Meeting the needs of our daily obligations can drain us, frustrate us, and slowly kill us in both body and spirit. If you wish to pursue spiritual growth and you lack the strength to devote to this goal, this book can help. With just a few minutes a day of dynamic movement and consciously controlled breathing, you will begin to move your Chi, or vital energy, and you will experience heightened levels of physical energy, greater mental clarity, and a more fit and flexible body. As your reservoir of energy increases, your joy in life will increase, you will possess a greater capacity to function happily and productively in your daily life, and your spiritual progress begins.

Energize! blends the esoteric traditions of yoga, sufism and taoism. You have the remarkable opportunity to learn Chinese *T'ai Chi Chi Kung, T'ai Chi Ruler,* and Red Dragon *Chi Kung;* East Indian Chakra Energizers; Middle Eastern Sufi Earth Dancing, Veil Dancing and Whirling; and the Native American Dance of the Four Directions, all at your own pace in the privacy of your own home.

0-87542-060-5, 240 pgs., 6 x 9, 96 illus., softcover **$10.00**

THE ART OF SPIRITUAL HEALING
by Keith Sherwood

Each of you has the potential to be a healer; to heal yourself and to become a channel for healing others. Healing energy is always flowing through you. Learn how to recognize and tap this incredible energy source. You do not need to be a victim of disease or poor health. Rid yourself of negativity and become a channel for positive healing.

Become acquainted with your three auras and learn how to recognize problems and heal them on a higher level before they become manifested in the physical body as disease.

Special techniques make this book a "breakthrough" to healing power, but you are also given a concise, easy-to-follow regimen of good health to follow in order to maintain a superior state of being. This is a practical guide to healing.

0-87542-720-0, 224 pgs., 5 ¼ x 8, illus., softcover   **$7.95**

MEDITATION & HUMAN GROWTH
A Practical Manual for Higher Consciousness
Genevieve Lewis Paulson

Meditation has many purposes—healing, past life awareness, balance, mental clarity and relaxation are just a few. Meditation & H8man Growth is a life-long guidebook that focuses on the practice of meditation as a tool for growth and development, as well as for expanding consciousness into other realms. It includes detailed meditations of both a "practical" and more esoteric nature to serve the needs of the complete person. Specific exercises are provided for different areas of life: health of the physical body; wealth in the physical world; emotional well-being; transmuting excess sexual energy; experiencing oneness with the universe; and alignment with the seasonal, lunar and planetary energies.

Meditation is a way of opening into areas that are beyond our normal thinking patterns. In fact, what we now call "altered states" and "peak experiences" will become the normal consciousness of the future. This book is full of techniques for those who wish to claim those higher vibrations and expanded awareness for their lives today.

0-87542-599-2, 224 pgs., 6 x 9, illus., softcover   **$12.95**

THE WOMEN'S BOOK OF HEALING
by Diane Stein

At the front of the women's spirituality movement with her previous books, Diane Stein now helps women (and men) reclaim their natural right to be healers. Included are exercises which can help YOU to become a healer! Learn about the uses of color, vibration, crystals and gems for healing. Learn about the auric energy field and the Chakras.

The book teaches alternative healing theory and techniques and combines them with crystal and gemstone healing, laying on of stones, psychic healing, laying on of hands, chakra work and aura work, and color therapy. It teaches beginning theory in the aura, chakras, colors, creative visualization, meditation, health theory and ethics with some quantum theory. Forty-six gemstones plus clear quartz crystals are discussed in detail, arranged by chakras and colors.

The Women's Book of Healing is a book designed to teach basic healing (Part I) and healing with crystals and gemstones (Part II). Part I discusses the aura and four bodies; the chakras; basic healing skills of creative visualization, meditation and color work; psychic healing; and laying on of hands. Part II begins with a chapter on clear quartz crystal, then enters gemstone work with introductory gemstone material. The remainder of the book discusses, in chakra-by-chakra format, specific gemstones for healing work, their properties and uses.

0-87542-759-6, 352 pgs., 6 x 9, illus., softcover $12.95

CHAKRA THERAPY
For Personal Growth & Healing
by Keith Sherwood

Understand yourself, know how your body and mind function and learn how to overcome negative programming so that you can become a free, healthy, self-fulfilled human being.

This book fills in the missing pieces of the human anatomy system left out by orthodox psychological models. It serves as a superb workbook. Within its pages are exercises and techniques designed to increase your level of energy, to transmute unhealthy frequencies of energy into healthy ones, to bring you back into balance and harmony with your self, your loved ones and the multidimensional world you live in. Finally, it will help bring you back into union with the universal field of energy and consciousness.

Chakra Therapy will teach you how to heal yourself by healing your energy system because it is actually energy in its myriad forms which determines a person's physical health, emotional health, mental health and level of consciousness.

0-87542-721-9, 256 pgs., 5 ¼ x 8, illus., softcover $7.95

16 STEPS TO HEALTH AND ENERGY
A Program of Color & Visual Meditation, Movement & Chakra Balance
by Pauline Wills & Theo. Gimble

Before an illness reaches your physical body, it has already been in your *auric* body for days, weeks, even months. By the time you *feel* sick, something in your life has been out of balance for a while. But why wait to get sick to get healthy? Follow the step-by-step techniques in *16 Steps to Health and Energy*, and you will open up the energy circuits of your subtle body so you are better able to stay balanced and vital in our highly toxic and stressful world.

Our subtle anatomy includes the "energy" body of 7 chakras that radiate the seven colors of the spectrum. Each chakra responds well to a particular combination of yoga postures and color visualizations, all of which are provided in this book.

At the end of the book is a series of 16 "workshops" that help you to travel through progressive stages of consciousness expansion and self-transformation. Each session deals with a particular color and all of its associated meditations, visualizations and yoga postures. Here is a truly holistic route to health at all levels! Includes 16 color plates!

0-87542-871-1, 224 pgs., 6 x 9, illus., softcover   **$12.95**

CREATE YOUR OWN JOY
A Guide for Transforming Your Life
by Elizabeth Jean Rogers

Uncover the wisdom, energy and love of your higher self and discover the peace and joy for which you yearn! This highly structured journal-workbook is designed to guide you through the process of understanding how you create your own joy by how you choose to respond to people and situations in your life.

Each chapter offers guided meditations on overcoming blocks—such as guilt, grief, fear and destructive behavior—that keep happiness from you; thoughtful questions to help you focus your feelings; concrete suggestions for action; and affirmations to help you define and fulfill your deepest desires and true needs. As you record your responses to the author's questions, you will transform this book into a personal expression of your own experience.

Life is too short to waste your energy on negative thoughts and emotions—use the uncomplicated, dynamic ideas in this book to get a fresh outlook on current challenges in your life, and open the door to your joyful higher self.

1-56718-354-9, 240 pgs., 6 x 9, illus., softcover   **$10.00**